How to find a Midwife and Doula, in the pursuit of a more natural childbirth experience

Petra Ortiz

DEDICATION

With immense love and gratitude for the diamonds
from my womb:

Eric, Adam, Bruno, Alex, Ethan

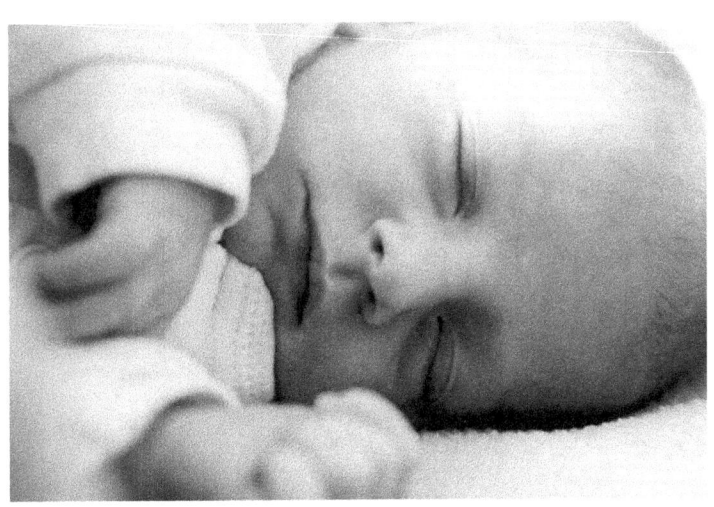

ACKNOWLEDGMENTS

I want to thank the contributing authors who were extremely cooperative and giving of their time, for providing valuable and refreshing content; I really appreciate you.

In addition, I wish to thank the photographers for their beautiful depictions, which help to create a rewarding experience for you, the Reader.

I would also like to thank Sam, Bruno and Carl for agreeing to my 'demand' to hire a midwife for each of our respective children; and for always being very loving and supportive of our sons. Mom-without your constant stories- I would have never embarked on trying to do this 'on my own'. So, I thank you as well.

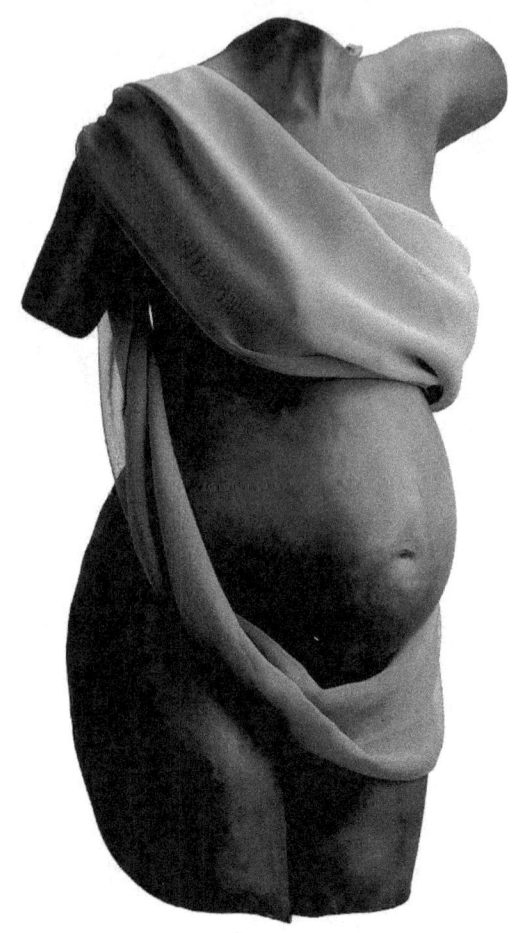

Introduction

In this book, you will learn what a Midwife is, and what a Doula is—and more importantly, what they can do for you, how they can support you, and how to locate either or both to discuss your pursuit of a natural childbirth. You are encouraged to locate and interview one or both, in your area after reading this work. You will learn what to expect from a Midwife or Doula during the prenatal, labor & delivery, and postpartum stages of your pregnancy, and receive heartfelt advice on your new 'job' as a parent. There is no doubt you will want to discuss where you would like to give birth [whether that be at your home, a hospital, or a birthing center (a medical center, but in a home-type setting), how to write your own birth plan, methods of pain relief, coping skills, nutrition needs and more. By interviewing, and gathering information from across the country [and UK] for this book, I hope that by the time you finish reading it, your top questions and concerns have been answered well, and that new ideas have manifested a feeling of empowerment in you.

Natural childbirth is loosely defined as labor and childbirth without medical intervention, meaning, that no drugs are given to relieve pain, nor aid in the birth process. It is considered the safest method for the baby, and is based on the notion that women who are adequately prepared, are able (innately) to give birth to their child, in an unrestricted manner; they are usually assisted by a Midwife and / or Doula. In my opinion, this is the only way that one can become 'adequately prepared'.

A Birth Plan is usually created during your visit, which lists what your wishes are for your actual delivery experience. It is a written list of your preferences to be used as a guide for how you would like your labor and delivery to 'go'. As labor can be unpredictable, you may need to deviate from this plan at times during labor. Your chosen Midwife or Doula can assist you with its creation.

The reason I wrote this book was because I wanted to provide a way for pregnant individuals (or couples) who are considering natural childbirth options, to be able locate a midwife and / or doula more easily, and know what to expect during the entire process (from the first interview to the postpartum stage) *before* actually embarking on that search. I also wanted to explain exactly what that support entails. Because they do in fact provide two different types of support for you (and your partner).

In short, I want you to be much more prepared than I was.

When I was first pregnant [in 1991], I knew I wanted to attempt a home birth, but I did not know how I was going to accomplish it, nor how to find a midwife to help me. All I knew was that I did not want to be rushed during labour, I wanted to be able to have people around me that I cared about as opposed to 'strangers', and I did not want to have an unnecessary Cesarean operation like my Mother endured [for many years, my Mom lamented about how her Doctor did not want to wait past a few hours of labour, and thus delivered me via vertical Cesarean cut; then performed the same operation down the same horrific (sorry Mom!) scar for my two siblings].

Nowadays, there are many more midwives and doulas to assist you. But if you have never called upon one for assistance, never had one help you deliver your baby, or provide pain relief options for you, or provide guidance and support for your partner-I hope that this book will help you make the decision to consider trying one or both. And I never ever want Dads to be left out. In fact, I wish that all Dads and Partners would want to be present and extra supportive during labour and delivery; so I have some special info for you in here too.

It is not important to relay my own birth stories here-because every person is different, thus every labour will be different. I am not a midwife, nor a doula; I am merely a messenger. With that, I hope you enjoy and benefit immensely from my contributing authors' information and guidance for you.

****

It is my sincere hope, wish and prayer that you come away being much more informed about your options, and looking forward to a natural birth, with anticipation and *trust in yourself.*

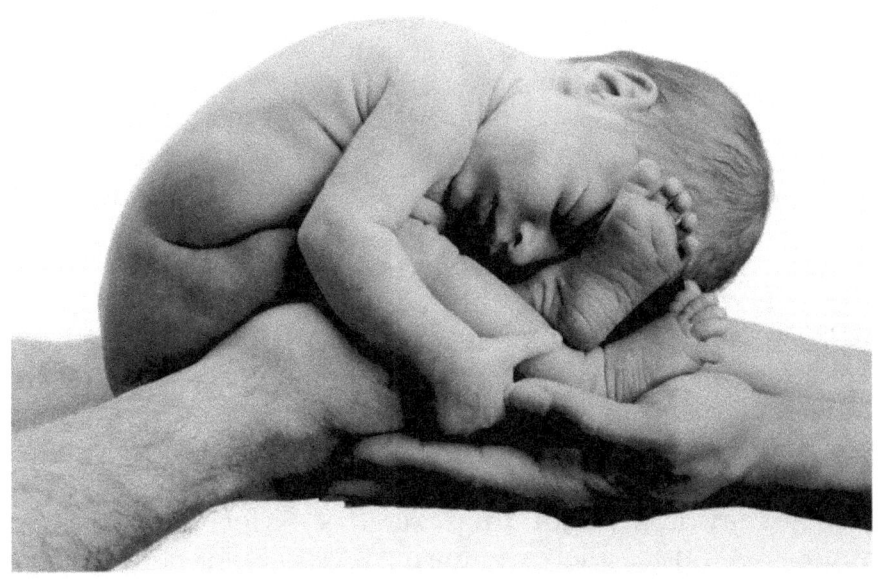

1 NATURAL BIRTH THE FIVE CRITICAL FACTORS

Keith Roberts

As a birth doula, I work entirely in a hospital setting, where I feel most needed, and where natural births are talked about but seldom seen. Over the past seventeen years that I have been assisting birthing families, five important factors have stood out as essential for having a natural birth. I will enlarge on these factors and explain their role, as we, as doulas, can have some influence over all five. First, allow me to define natural birth in a hospital setting: a mother in labor is admitted to the hospital and delivers her baby with nothing more than being monitored and possibly having the requisite IV [Intra Venous, administered into a vein, as an injection]. Although all women are not aiming for a natural childbirth, and we support the decisions each woman chooses, I find through my prenatal massage practice that the clear majority of pregnant mothers would like to have a natural birth, while the vast majority do not achieve it.

Why is there this enormous disparity?

Two short answers are fear and expectation – the mother's fear of the process, and a hospital-driven expectation of multiple and routine interventions. With this definition of natural birth, I believe mothers who achieve this remain below three percent (exclude the occasional precipitous birth delivered in triage in any hospital setting). Consider the high epidural [injection of anesthetic into the space outside the dura mater enveloping the spinal cord] rate (often above 90%), rising rates of cesarean births and inductions (without medical need) [the inducing of labor, whereby labor is initiated artificially with drugs, such as oxytocin], decreasing support of a trial of labor following a cesarean section (VBAC [vaginal birth after a cesarean birth]), and the trivializing of artificial rupture of membranes in early labor by doctors. I would also suggest that since hospitals charge handsomely for their myriad interventions (and surely budget against that income) that they have, in fact, a disincentive to lower the use of any of these services. Interventions have become the American way of doing the birth business in hospitals in this country.

So mothers who desire a natural birth have a system to buck and expectations to cast aside. I believe they must be proactive and assertive to achieve their goal, and I have some guides to follow – let's call them critical factors. What I believe to be the five critical factors in having a natural birth have not come from the writing of others, but from my experiences over the years in labor and delivery and through my prenatal massage practice. The critical factors are: education, choice of health care provider, retention of amniotic fluid, avoidance of an induction, and use of a doula.

Education

Education implies that a birthing couple will become knowledgeable about the whole birth process, with this important outcome: reduce fear. It should combine reading with a childbirth class, as well as seeking voices of positive expectation. This self-educating reduces the unknowns, thus bringing down fear. I like to tell mothers that, "We have complete trust that your body knows how to develop this baby. It's also true that your body knows how to give birth to this baby. There is nothing you have to figure out. Birth is all about letting go, and your job is to get out of the way. Trust the process." Trust is one side of a coin; the other side is fear. Ideally, as a birth doula, I want the mothers I work with to have a great trust in the process and little fear. And I know my very presence will be reassuring. This is a win/win coin.

Choice of Health Care Provider

The next critical factor in having a natural birth is choice of doctor. A couple needs to do some homework: talk to other birthing couples, develop a list of questions, and interview more than one obstetrician. One significant piece of information I would want to know would be the doctor's cesarean rate, for I believe this number reflects on his/her patience with birthing mothers and the process of labor and delivery. For more information on how to get transparency from your local hospitals and doctors, see www.thebirthsurvey.com

Over the past several years I've realized that all OB's fall somewhere along a continuum that falls between patient driven care to medical model or managed care. I would suggest natural birth occurs most often at the patient driven care end where the doctor is interested in the birth plan and promises to help the couple implement it. This doctor is also proud to announce his/her very low cesarean birth rate.

As you can guess, my favorite OB's are not in a hurry. Similar to midwives, they are on baby time and display trust in the process by being willing to wait rather than intervene where possible. Sometimes I feel body language says it all. Doctors broadcast their impatience in their movements, their choice of words, and the time/clock expectations they voice ("I'll be back in two hours, and I expect you to have dilated two centimeters by then."). Know that obstetricians need your business.

They may tell you what they think you want to hear. Talk specifically about birth without intervention and listen carefully to their responses. Any time they say, "We'll have to talk about that later (when you're in labor)", they're hedging and that's a red flag. Does he/she seem to be in a hurry in the interview? Yes? Don't expect it to be any different when you're in labor! Couples are really on their own here as they make this most important decision of provider. Now, they need to be patient. Interview some more. Of course my favorite providers are doula friendly and offer their pregnant mothers doula's names to call. Do you want a natural birth? Ask doulas who they recommend! Expect them to name OB's who practice like the midwifery model: preserve the amniotic fluid, largely ignore the clock, suggest no interventions to speed up the process when mother and baby are looking good, and support her birth plan to the extent possible. Also expect doulas to recommend midwives, for many of them embody the behaviors that stem from seeing birth as a natural process, with great patience and positive expectations.

Avoid an Induction
(for non-medical reasons)

The ever increasing rate of inductions is of great interest. In 1990 the induction rate was 9.5%. In 2003 it had risen to 28%, and in 2009 it was reported to be over 40% and rising. While these percentages vary slightly from source to source, they all point to an alarming upward trend. And three of four inductions are being performed without a clear medical need!

To the mother who wants a natural birth, I would say, "Wait to go into labor spontaneously. Yes, you're uncomfortable, but now you need to be patient." Just say 'no thank you' when your OB offers to induce you, "Next Monday, as that is the only day I'll be at the hospital in the next three weeks." Never mind that you are only a 6 or 7 on the Bishop's Scale and you will not have reached your due date by then [the Bishop's Scale is a sort of pre-labor scoring system to assist in predicting whether induction of labor will be required]. And don't let "due date" alone persuade you to be induced. Author, Henci Goer, in The Thinking Woman's Guide to a Better Birth, points out that the 40 week pregnancy was set in the early 1800's, and according to a 1990 study we should add 8 days to the calendar of a woman who is pregnant for the first time, and 3 days for mothers having their second baby. In fact, 41 weeks is the median length of pregnancy in healthy first-time mothers, meaning that one-half of these pregnancies will last longer than 41 weeks. If you and your baby are healthy and your blood pressure and amniotic fluid level are fine, let your baby mature in the uterus.

Hospital protocols for an induction can make it very hard to weather the pain from the hospital's standard interventions. In my area, Colorado Springs, the induction usually begins with Cytotec to soften the cervix. Cytotec, a drug prescribed for stomach ulcers, is being used in an off-label way, and carries the risk of uterine hyper-stimulation and fetal distress. The water is routinely broken with an accompanying dramatic shift in the level of pain. Pitocin is added to the IV line to cause contractions and is increased over time. Within an hour, the contractions usually start and increase in intensity as the dosing of Pitocin is raised. For the great majority of mothers the pain load prompts them to ask for an epidural. Their hope for a drug free, natural birth has been ruined. And for about 40% of them, they will end up with a cesarean section [the delivery of a fetus by surgical incision through the abdominal wall and uterus].

Induction carries risks of course. There is an increased risk of an abnormal fetal heart rate. Expect an increased use of forceps or vacuum extraction because when labor is induced, babies tend to stay in unfavorable positions. There is a greater probability that your baby will be admitted to the neonatal intensive care unit, with you being apart from your baby and with breastfeeding getting off to a poor start. Prematurity and jaundice are a greater risk, as well as increased risk of cesarean section.

These are sobering consequences from choosing to be induced without a medical need. Wait. Wait for your baby's sake and for yours. Patience is your greatest asset near full term and beyond!

Keep Your Water
In my area, artificial rupture of membranes (AROM) is routine upon admission to the hospital and trivialized as an intervention. The dialogue usually goes something like this: the obstetrician says, "I would like to check you, and I would like to break your water to speed things up a little bit." What isn't said is that in the next few minutes your pain will dramatically increase and you will be asking for the epidural. If she says nothing or consents, her plan for a natural birth has potentially been sabotaged.

The statement of the OB is very seductive. The implied promise is that labor will be shorter. There is no mention of the terrible trade-off in terms of increased pain and possible problems for the baby. I encourage my mothers to say, "No thank you. I am not in a hurry." When AROM becomes routine, medical need is not mentioned, as both mother and baby are doing fine. So I encourage my clients to keep their water and be ready to speak up on their own behalf, as I am not their voice. Keeping their water is something they should read and decide about before coming to the hospital.

Because of the pain factor, I think keeping the amniotic fluid as long as possible is crucial to having a natural birth – at least until eight or nine centimeters. Note too that an induction can be started without breaking the water. You can do it nicely, but just say, "No thank you" if you don't want the procedure.

Here are four compelling reasons to say, "Leave my water alone". First, the amniotic fluid that surrounds the baby also surrounds the cord. It is much less likely that the cord will become compressed if it is surrounded by the amniotic fluid. Take away the water and there may be decelerations on the monitor. The decels can be worrisome enough to begin an amnio infusion or send the client for a cesarean birth. Leave the water alone. Secondly, the amniotic fluid serves as a lubricant that allows the baby to twist and turn and descend. Take the water away, and the baby may get stuck. Stuck babies often go to cesarean birth. Leave the water alone. Thirdly, sometimes, late in labor, it may be discovered that the baby is poorly positioned. Perhaps the head is to the side or the baby's face is toward the front of mother's tummy. As doulas, we know to get a mother to lunge with a foot up on a chair, or get on hands and knees for an extended length of time (or any number of other remedies). And we expect the baby's position to become more favorable – if she still has her water. No water? No luck. Leave the water alone. And fourthly, of greatest immediate impact to the mother is the fact that her amniotic fluid serves as a wonderful buffer for pain. She may feel like contractions are a real challenge, but they are tolerable. That cushion of water is effective counter pressure. Leave the water alone.

Hire a Doula

With a natural birth rate in hospitals of an estimated 3% or less, most mothers have fallen victim to a system that lives by the clock, is ever ready to use their tools and inject their medicines, and is often in a hurry. Their expectations result from their daily experiences of natural birth being obstructed in countless ways. Now include the doula. Having assisted at 175 births, my natural birth rate is 71%, with nearly three-fourths of my mothers only being monitored and having an IV.

So a birth doula is often the agent that brings the other critical factors together. Having a doula is like bringing a childbirth education class to labor and delivery. Having a doula is key to lowering fear because doulas are a continuous and calming presence that makes a mother feel fully supported; thus she feels safe and can let go of fear. After my daughter's second wonderful birth experience (yes, I was her doula), we were discussing how well she had done and she responded, "You know, Dad, I was just never afraid." What an important statement! What an impact that made on her progress! And I say to couples when they ask me to assist them, "In inviting me to your birth, you have put trust in me and have already let go of a certain amount of fear." These are important dynamics that help her step aside to allow the baby to come down and meet its new parents.

A doula at the birth can help with fetal positioning – or re-positioning – especially if the mother still has her water. It has been my experience that some providers will give a mother more time to labor, not even suggest AROM, use less interventions and demonstrate more trust in the process with a doula present that they like and respect. And we doulas have all come away from a natural birth in which we knew our emotional and physical support was the favorable, deciding factor. We helped that mother dig deep and she rose to the occasion; she surprised even herself and was euphoric over the outcome and extremely proud of herself. Yes, and all of that courage and satisfaction ultimately enhanced by bonding and breastfeeding.

For many mothers in my prenatal massage practice, I have been the first person to suggest that they could have a birth without narcotics or an epidural. Due to their fears they hadn't really entertained such a possibility. True, a natural birth was their desire; they just hadn't see themselves in that picture. There is an opportunity here for every doula to say, "You can do it too. We can do it together." Your voice may well be the first one to give her the courage to try. Ask her to talk about her fears, and let her know how your participation can be the all-important support she needs to meet her goal. I see every birth as being like a game of cards. The families will be dealt some good cards and perhaps some bad cards.

Whatever the hand, they have to play it. And as doulas our job is to help them play the hand well. Our experience helps us see the bigger picture and helps the couple navigate the system. Additionally, we can tailor our support to allow the husband or partner to also rise to the occasion, follow our lead, and become the strong emotional supporter he/she is surely capable of being. In the end, we have facilitated the natural birth and allowed the father/partner to shine. I call this doula magic.

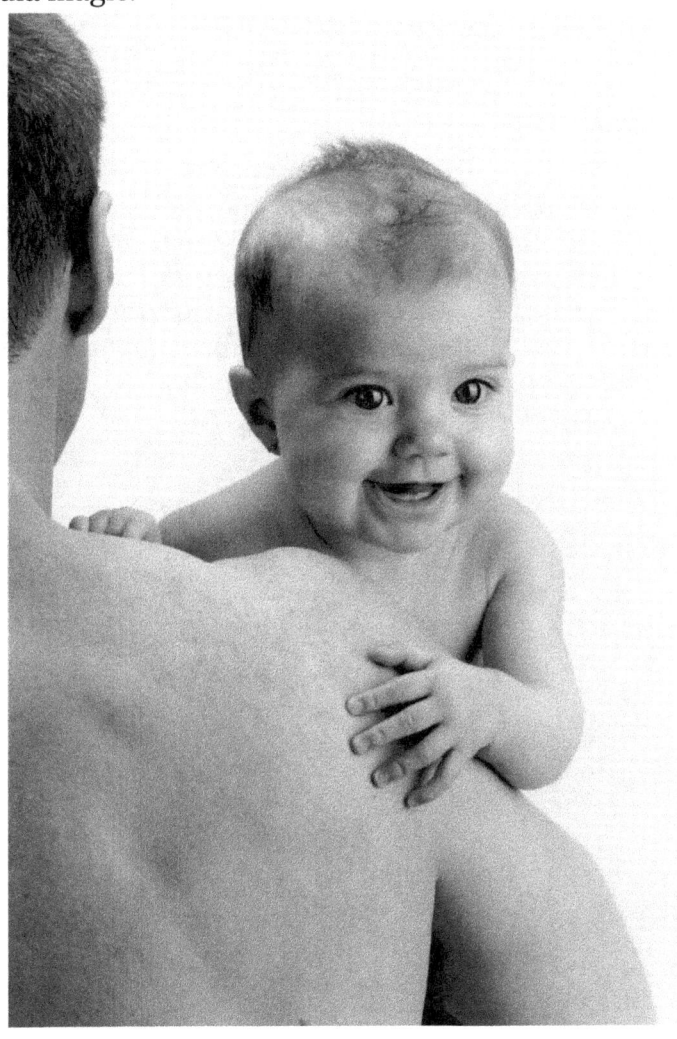

Which of these five critical factors is the most important? Can they be ranked in a 1-5 order? No, they are of equal importance. In their own way, each is crucial. It is up to each of us as doulas to continue to hone our skills, attend national conferences, cultivate relationships of acceptance and respect with providers, and garner sterling reputations as valuable and effective contributors, in our own right, to mothers and fathers during birth. Let us nurture ourselves as we continue to be the catalyst that allows a natural birth in a hospital setting. Let us continue to deliver our very own magic.

Keith Roberts is a full-time prenatal massage therapist in Colorado Springs, having worked on more than 1,100 mothers in the past 17 years. He is a DONA certified birth doula and has assisted at 175 births. He is also a studio photographer, photographing pregnant mothers and couples with their newborns. Many of his black and white prints are displayed in labor and delivery at local hospitals and OB offices. His photographs are included in this book in Chapters 1, 2 and 4.

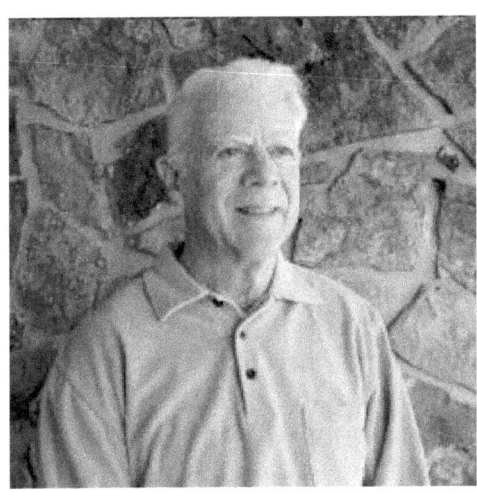

2 DOULA MAGIC

Keith Roberts

How do you view birth / What is your philosopy?
Because I live in the United States and work as a birth doula here, I see birth as a highly medicalized experience. For mothers who want a natural birth, with no interventions, it is a hard system to buck. From the very beginning, I realized that most OB's are in a hurry – not for the safety of mother or baby – but to somehow make the mother fit into their own schedule (with a few wonderful OB exceptions who are clearly on "baby time"). The message to parents is to choose your doctor wisely. The "baby time" OB practices like a midwife, with great patience. If your obstetrician is in a hurry with prenatal visits, it won't be any different in labor and delivery. Ask birth doulas who they like to work with.

Why did you decide to become a Doula?
I became a birth doula as my life unfolded after retiring from 31 years as a classroom teacher. I went to massage school a year before I retired and became a licensed massage therapist in 1995. At that same time, my wife began taking silversmithing lessons. Her instructor came to me for massages. When she got pregnant, she continued to see me.

We both realized that the work I did on her helped relieve her hip and low back pain and helped her mobility.

Within a week of her delivery, I received a course offering in the mail to become certified in prenatal massage. It was a very thorough training and I earned that certification in 1996. I heard the word "doula" for the first time. I decided to specialize in pregnancy massage and soon felt I had found my calling. Over the next two years I followed fifteen of my prenatal massage clients into labor and delivery. I focused on physical support, applying sacral counter pressure with contractions and using hot towels on the low back between contractions. I realized I was making a significant difference during the birthing experience as mother after mother needed no pain medication. I decided that I needed to become a certified birth doula, as that was exactly what I was doing.

My favorite part of being a doula is watching mothers and fathers fall in love with their new son or daughter. How often in life do we get to watch someone fall in love? I don't usually get teary at a birth unless the father cries. Now that is special. I have seen many fathers (and mothers) wipe away tears as they hold their newborn -- powerful stuff. It's such a privilege to witness this.

I went through doula training with Doulas of North America and received that certification in 2000. Along with my certificate was a handwritten note that said that I was the first male to be certified with Doulas of North America. I was number 1303.

Keith,

I am writing to let you know that you are officially a DONA certified doula! Congratulations! You will be receiving paperwork within about 4 weeks or so. You can however, begin using CD (DONA) now.

You have the unique distinction of being the first male doula we have ever certified. Your packet was wonderful, and it is obvious that the families you support are very lucky. Thank you for all your efforts.

In the doula spirit,
J. Swann
DONA Certification Chair

Currently I have done massage on over 1,100 pregnant mothers and have assisted at 175 hospital births (including my daughters' two children), and counting...and I certainly have a short list of my favorite, very patient OB's.

What are your certifications and what do they mean?

I am a licensed massage therapist, registered with the state of Colorado (1995). I am certified in prenatal massage, so I have special training to meet the needs of pregnant mothers throughout their pregnancy and beyond (1996). This is my full time massage specialty. I am also a certified birth doula with Doulas of North America (2000). I work wholly in the hospital setting where I feel I am most needed.

What should a client expect from you during the prenatal stage?

During the prenatal stage, I often see doula clients for several pregnancy massages where I focus on the hips and low back during 90 minute sessions. I always stretch the low back at the end of the massage with a procedure called pelvic stabilization, which gives stretch to the quadratus lumborum at the top of the pelvis at the illiac crest. The QL typically gets tight and is painful as these two muscles at the level of the waist shorten to help stabilize mother's posture as she gets bigger and her center of gravity shifts forward. This massage work improves mobility throughout pregnancy as pain is reduced.

Toward the end of the prenatal stage I have a two hour meeting at 36/37 weeks to help prepare the couple for labor and delivery. It is a time to talk about what to expect in more detail, to answer questions and for the couple to take notes. I offer several suggestions for the birth plan. Then we go into my massage studio to practice the pushing stage for the sake of positioning, breathing and pacing. We rehearse pushing on my massage table in the semi-lithotomy position (lying on her back) as well as in side lying. This practice prepares the father to know what to do when his wife says, "I need to push." It is a great confidence builder for the dad who may well be going down this birthing road for the first time. During this couple meeting, I also teach the father how to do counter pressure on the sacrum during contractions. We practice with the mother saying "starting" and "easing". Dad can do counter pressure at home when his wife is in early labor. I show several ways to incorporate the birth ball into her labor. And finally I show the couple how they can use their own crock pot as a towel heater and how to safely apply a hot, wet towel to her sacrum between contractions at home. I believe partners can do effective physical support at home. At the hospital I take over that kind of support so that Dad can move into the role of emotional supporter, as that is where the intimacy is.

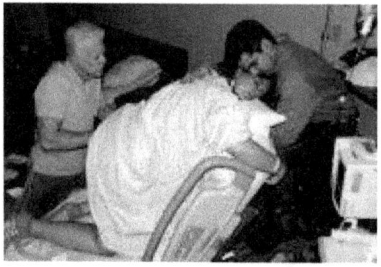

In this photo, Keith is applying sacral counter pressure to a woman who is in labor with her third child; she is sitting on a birth ball. This is his third birthing experience with this couple.

As a birth doula I focus equally on both parents and I work hard to enable the husband to assist his partner at the level he is comfortable with. I help him help her. Ultimately I hope the father will rise to the occasion and be the strong emotional mainstay and shoulder to lean on. His wife will want to look into his eyes and hold his hand. I want him to shine and be remembered for his unique contributions to her birthing experience. And in my experience over the years, I have seen many fathers do a magnificent job, just given the chance.

What should a Client expect from you during labor and delivery stages?

During labor and delivery I focus on strong physical support by applying about 35 pounds of counter pressure on the sacrum during every contraction and by applying a hot, wet towel to the mother's low back between contractions. The birth partner will also be a focal point, as I want to help him to be involved as the most important emotional supporter. To the extent that he takes on that role, I am thrilled because there is a need for touching and intimacy that he can fulfill if given the chance.

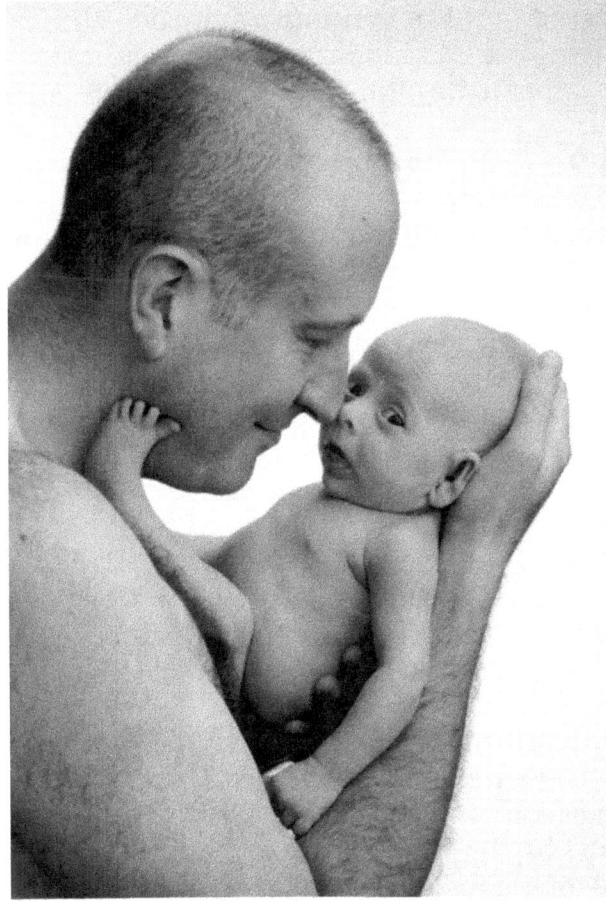

When the mother begins to push, we each take a leg and help her open her pelvis. We have rehearsed this in my massage studio, and now it's time to apply the lesson. This is another opportunity for the father to be completely involved and to witness the birth of his child.

As a birth doula I feel it is up to me to reserve tasks for the father in which he can shine and to keep he and his wife connected as much as possible. She will want to see his face, hold his hand and hear his voice. I save this space for him.

Having a doula at your birth is like taking your childbirth class with you into labor and delivery. As doulas we interpret what is going on, give perspective in a positive way and we can give advice if asked. So I am an important source of information which can serve as a calming influence and can continually enable the father to be intimately and effectively engaged.

What should a client expect from you during the postpartum stage?

Due to my gender difference, I do not serve as a lactation consultant. I have a lot of information regarding nursing, but this is a line I have chosen not to cross. I always go back to the hospital to visit the next day and I get to hold the baby! I also deliver insurance paperwork the couple can send into their insurance company to seek full reimbursement for my services. And some mothers come back to me for postpartum massage, as I am trained in that area as well. Additionally many couples bring their newborn to my photo studio for photographs. I still am using film which I develop in my darkroom and make handmade prints to keep that tradition alive. All my work is in beautiful black and white. And I have a following of people who want exactly that.

What questions do you typically ask when interviewing a prospective client?

My first question is always, "What kind of birth experience do you want?" I begin this way because I am bound by my code of ethics and my standards of practice with Doulas of North

America to support the kind of birth the couple aspires to have. The vast majority who seek me out say they want a natural birth without medication.

In that case I believe they are right to hire a doula, for we bring tools of the heart and hands that encourage courage and give enough pain relief through counter pressure and heat on the low back that help a determined mother to dig deeply to accomplish the natural birth she so desires. So often I have seen women powerfully rise to the occasion and labor one contraction at a time to finally deliver their baby free from any pain medication or other interventions. And just as often it was the doula's unwavering emotional and physical support that raised the bar of expectation and kept saying, "You can do this." The mother, in turn voices, "I can do this," and she does. And the staff gets to witness another powerful woman having a powerful birth experience.

For those who say they want an epidural as soon as possible, I will support that as well. And sometimes, with the continuous help of a doula, the labor progresses and the mother realizes that while it is challenging, she is doing ok and delivers without any interventions. These deliveries are always followed by a great sense of pride and gratitude for having had a birth doula.

Of interest, 72 of my first 100 mothers delivered in a hospital with no interventions, other than being on a monitor and having the requisite IV. Read my article on "The Role of Expectation at Natural Births", published in International Doula magazine and included here in chapter 4.

What are common misconceptions you hear from prospective parent(s)?
The most common misconception that I hear is the idea that the water has to break for you to begin labor and make progress. And doctors often trivialize keeping the amniotic fluid by saying, "I would like to check you, and I would like to break your water to speed things up a bit." This is a rather

seductive statement, because it implies that we get to see the baby sooner – never mind the unspoken consequence of breaking the water without a clear medical reason. The mother can answer, "No thank you. I am not in a hurry." She did not give permission. The doctor made his statement knowing full well that in the next few minutes, there will be a dramatic shift in the level of pain and the mother will say, "I can't do this. Give me the epidural." If she wanted a natural birth, it was just sabotaged.

So I talk about this important issue at our couple meeting, and I let them know that it must be one of their voices that says, "No thank you. I am not in a hurry." The doula is not their voice at the hospital. I encourage all my mothers to keep their water as long as possible and let it break on its own. I ask them to read about it on their own and decide before they go to the hospital what they want in regard to retaining their amniotic fluid. If they decide to keep it, they must be prepared to speak up and defend it. Read my article on "Natural Birth: The Five Critical Factors" which is included here.

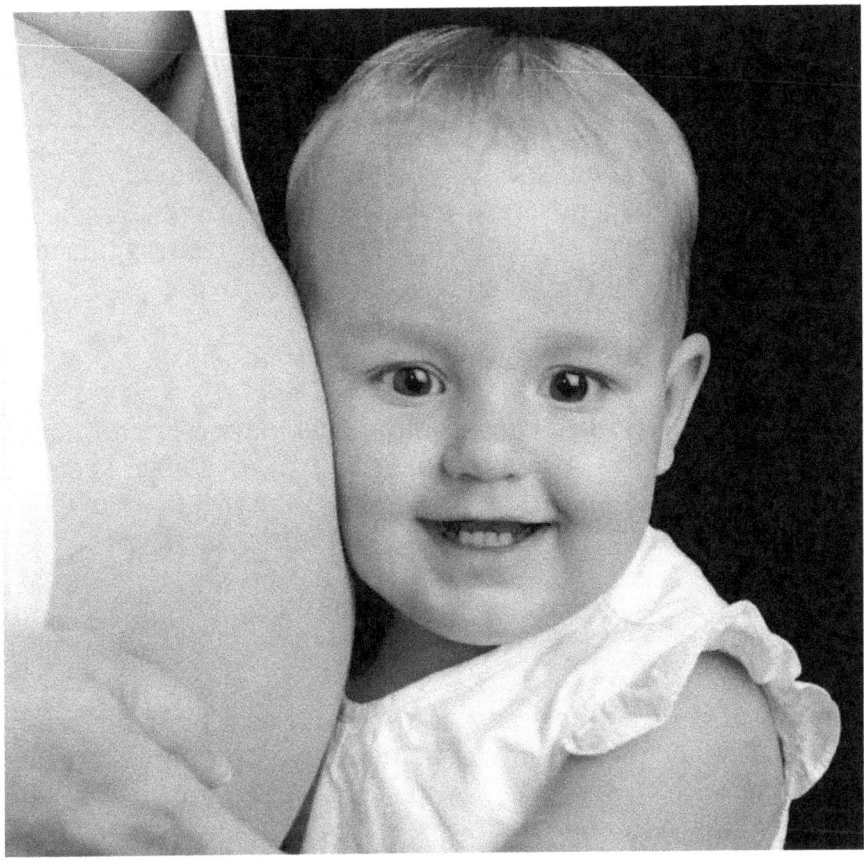

What are common questions you hear, and how do you answer those?

When should we go to the hospital? My advice begins: Expect to go into labor at night because you are a mammal. Observe early contractions. Eat a good supper, as you will not be fed in the hospital (You wouldn't begin a trip without filling the tank). Then go to sleep. As contractions get stronger you can time them. Wait until they are three minutes apart, they last one minute, and that has been going on for an hour. Also wait until you are in the second emotional stage of labor, as described by Dr. Robert Bradley. This is the "serious" stage, and it is marked by your not being able to answer a question until your contraction is over. So, eat a meal, progress to a 3,1,1 [as stated above: contractions that are three minutes apart, they last one minute and continue for an hour], and wait until you are in the "serious" emotional stage. Oh, and there may be one more signpost...you feel that you have lost all of your modesty.

A second common question: *What do I do if my water breaks at home?* It depends...are you Group B Strep [A type of streptococcal bacteria that when present in the vagina can cause problems for the baby] positive or negative?

If you are GBS positive, I would go on into the hospital.

But... if you are GBS negative, does the water have an odor? No. Is it clear? Yes. Then I would say hydrate and go to sleep. We'll talk in the morning. If you can't sleep, take your temperature every hour to confirm that it is not rising.

But if the water has an odor and/or has meconium...go on into the hospital.

Know that contractions may or may not begin after the water breaks. And the water breaking may be only a trickle. Continue to hydrate. Or if you feel uneasy, go on into the hospital. It's your call. In any case, I will meet you there.

What is the single most important advice you wish to give new parents? Established parents?

My single most important advice is to keep the amniotic fluid as long as possible if you want to have a natural birth. It serves as a wonderful buffer for pain, and I wouldn't give it up easily.

Secondly, I council couples to avoid an induction without a genuine medical reason. The rate of inductions is rapidly rising and four in ten will end in Cesarean Section. Induction for convenience is ill advised.

All of my most important advice is spelled out in my article: "Natural Birth: The Five Critical Factors".

What is your most memorable birthing experience?

My most memorable birth experiences are always those wherein the laboring mother digs deeply and says "I can do this" and she becomes the powerful woman she is and births without any interventions other than being monitored and having an IV. In attending 175 births, and counting, over the past 17 years, I have a whole new respect for the power of women!

What are some memorable references / letters of gratitude you would like to share here?

I received the following thank you note after a very long labor with a first time mother, who delivered on December 1, 2011:

Dear Keith

Words cannot express our deep gratitude for your unbelievable support in bringing our precious Ellie Rose into the world. Your knowledge, patience, love and encouragement gave us the tools and strength during our labor. We were able to have a labor full of grace – even during some very painful contractions!! We hope that you will be in our life for a very long time... hopefully you will be a doula for us again with our next baby?

With much gratitude,

Jackie and Jeff

What other services do you offer?

In addition to being a certified birth doula with Doulas of North America, I am a full time prenatal massage specialist, having worked on more than 1,100 mothers to date.

I am a studio photographer, and I take photos of pregnant mothers and families with newborns on film in black and white. Handmade prints are made in my darkroom.

How can someone learn more about your services, and contact you?

I may be reached via email at keithandjane@q.com and you may also learn more at my website www.keithrobertslmt.com

My phone number is listed there. Feel free to call me for more information about my birth services, or just to chat...

What organizations and / or websites do you recommend?

The easiest way to find a doula in your area is to go to www.DONA.org to find the Doulas of North America website.

Click on "Find a Doula", find your state, and there will be a list by cities of doulas who are certified by DONA.

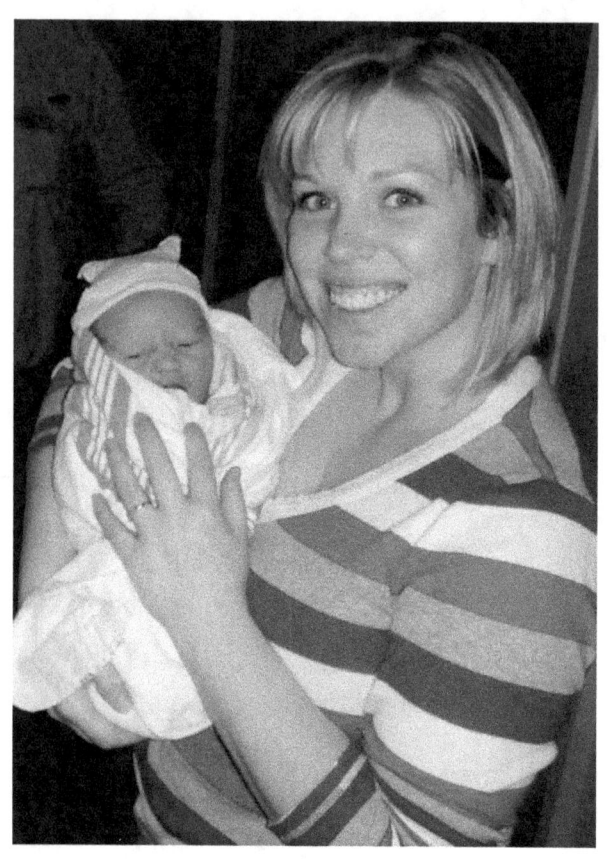

3 YOU HAVE A CHOICE

Kelly Burnett

How do you view birth / What is your philosophy?
I believe that birthing is a normal, natural occurring event in a woman's life and she deserves the support to do it HER own way.

Why did you decide to become a doula?
I decided to become a doula because of my own birthing experiences. My first pregnancy I was very uneducated about birth so I went into the hospital not knowing what to expect. I was induced, I was scared and the staff wasn't very nice. I was very glad to come out of the hospital not having a cesarean but

knew there was a lot that didn't seem quite right. I learned the most with my third child. I had a planned homebirth with two Certified Professional Midwives present and better yet, I did it! It is very important to me to help other women know they have choices and to educate them. Birth doesn't have to be something that you are afraid of.

What are your certifications and what do they mean?

I am in the process of certifying through Childbirth International.

What should a client expect from you during the prenatal stage?

I prefer we arrange two prenatal meetings before labor begins, preferably before 37 weeks in your pregnancy. Additional meetings may be arranged if necessary. This meeting gives us a chance to talk in detail about your preferences regarding your birth. If you have a Birth Plan, we will review it carefully. If you do not have a Birth Plan and would like to create one, I can assist with this.

I will want to know your own personal ways of coping with pain and fatigue and difficult situations, and what internal resources we can draw upon to assist you with the birthing experience. I will want to know how you and your partner foresee working together, and the roles of others who may be attending the birth. We can discuss together what fears and concerns you have regarding the birth. We can review your preferences regarding the use of pain medications. My role is to help you have a satisfying birth as you define it. The more we explore this in advance, the better I will be able to fulfill this role. This contract will be signed at or before the first prenatal meeting. I will also have informational handouts.

What should a client expect from you during labor and delivery stages?

During labor I will be there to support (emotionally and informationally), encourage and comfort her.

What should a client expect from you during the postpartum stage?

I usually remain for 1-2 hours after birth, until the mother is comfortable and the family is ready for quiet time together. I can also help with initial breastfeeding, if necessary. Also, about two days after the birth, we will have a postpartum visit where we can talk about her birth experience.

What questions do you typically ask when interviewing a prospective client?

I don't interview clients, they interview me to see if I am a good match for them. Once they have hired me I ask their due date, previous birth history, fears and concerns, and how do they think I can help them the most during labor, etc.

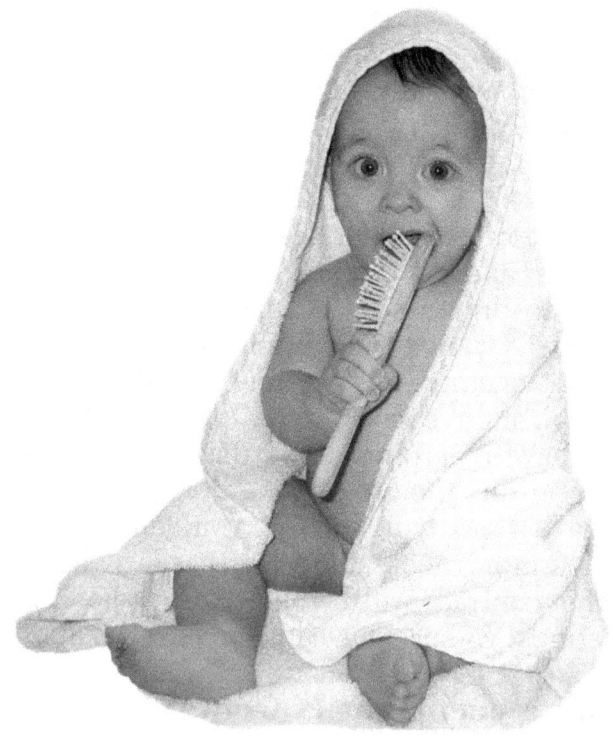

What are common misconceptions you hear from prospective parent(s)?

I have really bad heartburn, so my child will be born with lots of hair. (Pregnancy Myth)

This I find funny because I had been asked that A LOT!!! All three of my children were born with so much hair. My son had his first hair cut at two weeks!!!

You really get the pregnancy-induced heartburn because your baby is growing and your stomach is being pushed higher and whatever you eat, the acid moves backwards from the stomach to your lower esophagus irritating it and causing heartburn.

What are common questions you hear, and how do you answer those questions?

Most of the questions I hear are about the role of a doula, what is a doula, and why did I decide to become a doula. (Common Questions)

I explain that a doula is a person who provides support to women before, during and just after birth, and tell them why I became a doula.

What is the single most important advice you wish to give new parents? Established parents?

The most important thing I would say to new parents would be, sleep when the baby sleeps. To established parents, I would advise them to take time for themselves, quality time away from your child is just as important as quality time with your child.

What is your most memorable birthing experience?

My most memorable birthing experience is being able to be there for my sister and support her through pregnancy, practice labor (false labor), and birth. It was so much fun and exciting to share that with my best friend.

What other services do you offer?

At this time I don't offer any other service than birth doula service.

How can someone learn more about your services and contact you?

www.kellyburnettdoula.com
payingit4wrd@yahoo.com
423-385-0713

What is the fastest easiest way for a client to locate a doula?
www.Doulamatch.net and www.findadoula.com

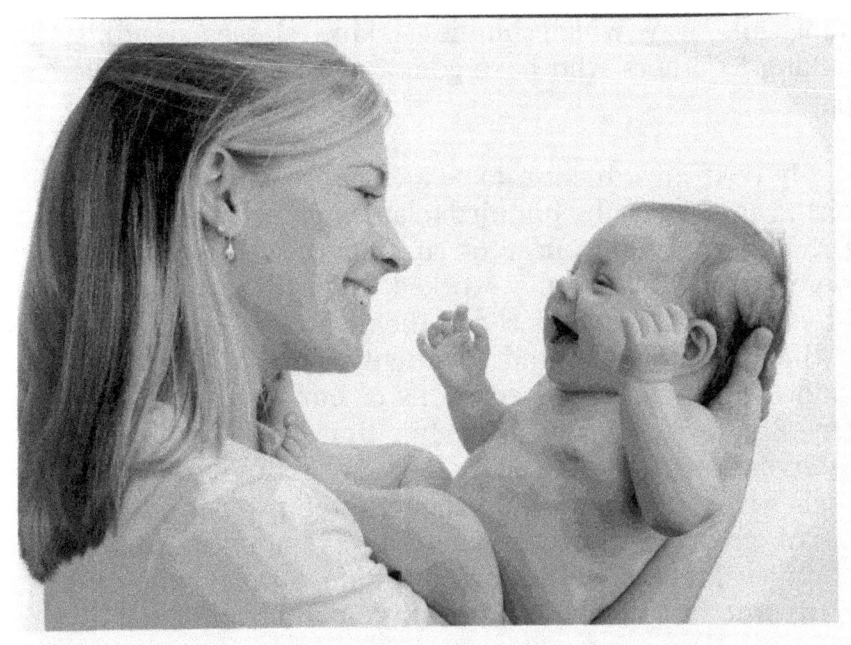

4 THE ROLE OF EXPECTATION AT NATURAL BIRTHS

Keith Roberts

Cover story of International Doula Magazine

in Volume 15, Issue 3, 2007

At every prenatal couple meeting, I make it clear that I will support the kind of birth experience this couple desires -- and I mean that. For those who aspire to a non medicated birth, I will offer ideas that I believe will facilitate that outcome. This article is an outgrowth of many years spent as a birth doula, helping make natural birth a satisfying reality.

Over the past twelve years that I have been assisting birthing mothers in a hospital setting, an important dynamic has emerged for me: the role of expectation as it applies to natural birth and doula support. Having a natural birth takes preparation; there are many important choices to be made along the way which implies taking classes, reading, and talking to others who have gone down this often challenging path.

My own introduction to -- and appreciation for -- natural birth came through childbirth classes my wife and I took with Dr. Robert Bradley in 1967 and 1970, when our daughters were born. Dr. Bradley worked to instill trust in the birth process; it was his underlying theme around which he helped us build confidence, and eventually our trust in the process guided our positive expectations of our own birth outcomes. Dr. Bradley was ahead of his time in shunning routine interventions, advocating fathers be allowed to accompany their wives into labor and expecting the partner's presence to be of great supportive value to his laboring mate. The "Bradley Method" continues to guide couples who trust the birth process and who need education and confidence.

I define "natural birth" in a hospital setting as a laboring mother having nothing more than electronic fetal monitoring and an IV after being admitted at four or five centimeters.

My guess is that actually happens in our hospitals less than five percent of the time (although much of the labor and delivery staff I have talked to here in Colorado Springs believe it to be under 3%.) Are you surprised? Well, take away the 70% to 90% of mothers who have epidurals, the 30% C-section rate, declining VBACs, and IV narcotics. Add in inductions, early rupture of membranes at admission, nurses encouraging drugs, doctors in a hurry, and horror stories freely told by other mothers. How many mothers are left who are laboring with confidence, on their way to a natural birth experience? (Allow me to quickly acknowledge the precipitous births of mothers admitting at eight or more centimeters and delivering in the next few minutes). The number of mothers left, who could possibly have an unmedicated birth, form a very small group indeed.

As you can see, we have a lot of fear-based "expectation" to overcome. I am a full time, prenatal massage therapist, and the vast majority of the nearly 900 mothers, who have come through my practice, would like to have a natural birth experience with no interventions. So where is the disconnect that facilitates the early AROMs, IV narcotics, epidurals and C-sections? I believe the disconnect is mother, nurse and doctor driven: by mothers through fear, nurses by daily experience, and doctors through being in a hurry.

For many new mothers, fear is acquired from listening to other mothers. And with our current, highly-medicalized hospital birth practices, mothers with bad experiences become the vocal majority -- and they are happy to share their stories. They usually advise, "Get the epidural". And the new mother, having heard from several of these women, promptly voices, "I will probably need/get an epidural." This has become her expectation. Doulas who strongly encourage and support natural birth have to start right here by providing a different vision, offering new possibilities and changing expectations.

Setting The Expectation With The Mother/Couple

Again, I see this as a given: most mothers want a natural birth; most expect to ask for an epidural. In interviews I always want to know what kind of birth experience the couple would like to have. If they aspire to a natural birth/pain medication-free birth, I can effectively support that. We will talk first about their trust in the process. And I listen carefully to their fears. I talk about trust and fear as being two sides of the same coin.

"You have complete trust that your body knows how to develop this baby, and you can have complete trust that your body knows how to birth this baby. TRUST this process." On the other side of the coin is fear; enter the doula. "When you have a doula at your birth, you will have someone who is a continuous presence; you will feel fully supported. And when you feel fully supported, you feel safe. Feeling safe allows you to let go of fear." There you have it: a high level of trust and a low level of fear. This is doula magic! Above all, as doulas, we can lower fear and enhance the process.

This is my beginning point in planting the seeds of great expectations. This may well be the first time someone has suggested that, "You can have a natural birth, and we can do this together." Many times I have felt a shift in attitude; it came from my positive voice and my own confidence. A mother must truly feel safe to really adopt our positive view, so our language is important, for it conveys our trust in the process. Our calmness in labor and delivery conveys our lack of fear.

I believe that a mother who feels empowered to embark on the natural birth journey should have this statement as the first one in her birth plan: "We would like to work with a nurse who is supportive of natural birth." We have set an expectation. Over the years I have been aware that this statement, along with the presence of a doula, can change a nurse's expectation. So many times I have heard, "Oh, you have Keith with you. You're going to have a wonderful birth." Substitute your own name for mine. You know the story. You have earned this reputation through hard work: sacral counter pressure, hot packs on the low back, movement, position changes, the shower, the birth ball, and a calm presence that speaks of trust in the process.

Nurses And Doctors Come On Board

A laboring mother's trust may inspire her to say, "I can do this," and labor accordingly. Nurses are sensitive to mothers who are succeeding with their coping skills, and they often become supportive in a different way. Their behavior changes; their language changes, and they too may adopt the natural birth goal of the mother. With all this positive energy the doctor can feel comfortable coming on board and allowing a natural birth to take place. I say allowing because doctors, too, may follow the lead of a mother laboring calmly with confidence and the support of her team.

One of the most striking behavior changes I have seen is that of giving a mother more time. This is no small relinquishment of control for take-charge doctors. But having trust in a doula (built over time) can put a mother in a different category. In this category there is a continuous presence of a competent doula, known to be patient and skilled in pain relieving comfort measures such as sacral counter pressure and hot packs on the low back. From past experience with this doula, the doctor knows this mother need not be labeled "failure to progress"; there is an expectation and a comfortability that allows more time to be given. We have all rejoiced at the end of a long labor with a vaginal birth; we were given more time, and we knew we made the difference. And doubtless, the doctor knew it too. Along with positive expectation, there must also be trust: trust in the process and trust in the doula. I recently assisted a VBAC mother who was allowed intermittent monitoring. I have worked with this OB several times before and have had powerful, natural birth outcomes.

This type of monitoring gave us the opportunity to change positions often, spending a lot of her time on hands and knees. The sacral pain focused in the low back changed to pubic pain focused in the front. What may have been an OP positioning [baby is head-down but facing your abdomen, the Occiput Posterior position] was obviously OA [Occiput Anterior, the ideal position for baby to pass through the pelvis; baby will be facing the mother's back with his back to one side of the mother's abdomen] at birth; what could have been a repeat C-section was a successful vaginal birth with no complications.

It is so much easier to try a variety of positions when not on the monitor.

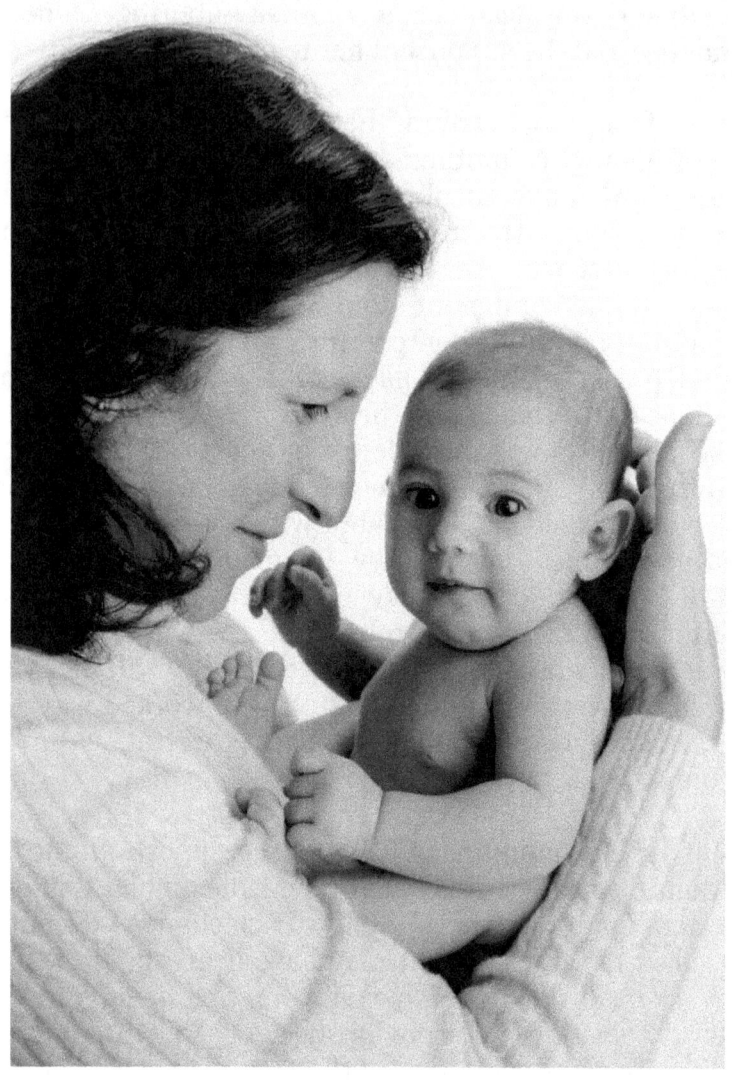

Keep Your Water: A Natural Aid to a Natural Birth

If a mother is determined to have a med-free birth experience, I want her to also be determined to keep her water. As doulas, if we have helped her to adopt the expectation that "I can do this", we must also help her understand how an early rupture of membranes can sabotage her aspirations. I want her to read about it and decide for herself about early rupture before she goes into labor. Henci Goer in "The Thinking

Woman's Guide to a Better Birth" addresses this well in Chapter 6 (subtitled: "If It Ain't Broke, Don't Break It"). In visiting childbirth education classes, I talk about what I see as the five critical factors in having a natural birth. Keeping the amniotic fluid is one of the five. The water serves as a highly effective buffer for pain and can be kept as long as possible for the sake of coping with the intensity of contractions.

When the doctor says, "I'd like to break your water to speed things up a little bit," the laboring mother can say, "No thank you. I'm not in a hurry." At a prenatal couple meeting I advise a couple to respond this way to the proposed AROM to preserve this all important pain cushion to avoid pain medications (all of which cross the placenta). Note that whatever has entered the baby's blood stream is trapped there the moment the cord is cut and has to be detoxified by the newborn.

We have all heard a mother say, "I can't do this" ten to fifteen minutes after the early rupture and request the epidural. "I plan to keep my water and let it break on its own" is an important statement in the birth plan.

While I see this issue often trivialized by doctors and nurses alike, I feel strongly that a mother retaining her water through full dilation is ideal, and it is a key component in achieving a natural birth.

I will soon have a "three-peat" with this doctor, with a mother whose first two births were memorable because of her confidence and determination. She needed no drugs, and she had the continuous support of a doula. The first question asked by her OB was... "Will you have Keith at your birth again?" Expectation: this mother/father-doula team will create another remarkable, natural birth. My expectation is that the behavior of the nurse and this OB will fully support our efforts, and we will all celebrate another birth without interventions.

While we have explored the influential role of expectation surrounding the birth process, positive expectation, and very possibly a new vision, are developed jointly with the couple and the doula. As they move into the hospital setting, the behavior of nurses and doctors may make subtle to dramatic changes that support this mother's natural birth goal. Let me stress that the doula must have earned respect at all levels. There is trust and confidence in this person, won over time through powerful birth experiences.

Every time you leave a birth and know you made a difference, you have also affected the complex of expectations that will go before you at your next birth. The role of expectation and the way it can change behavior is an extraordinary dynamic; it's doula magic!

Keith Roberts is a full-time prenatal massage therapist in Colorado Springs, having worked on over 1,100 mothers in the past 17 years. He is a DONA certified birth doula and has assisted at 175 births. He is also a studio photographer, photographing pregnant mothers and couples with their newborns. Many of his black and white prints are displayed in labor and delivery at local hospitals and OB offices. You can visit his website at www.KeithRobertsLMT.com and you may email him at keithandjane@q.com

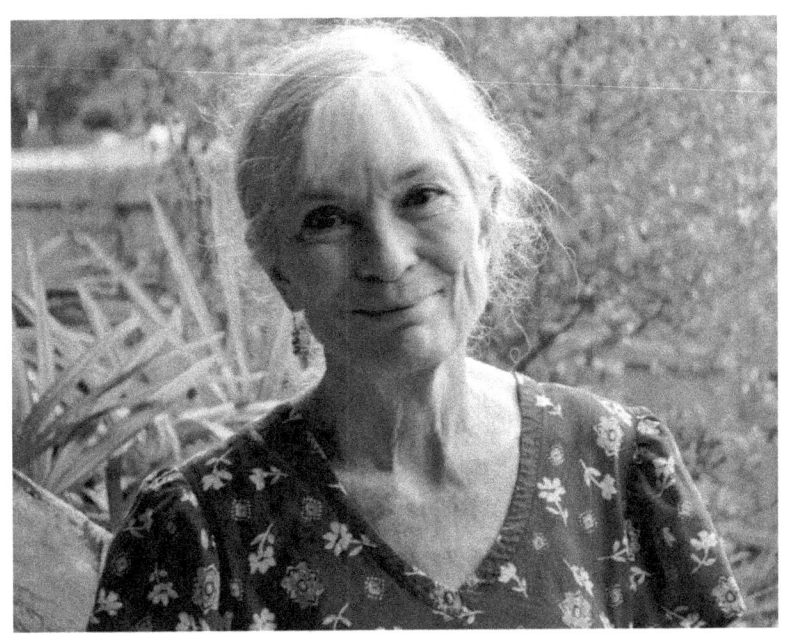

5 THE NEEDS OF THE MOTHER

Cathy Matthews

How do you view birth / What is your philosophy?
Birth is normally not a medical event, sometimes needing to be assisted in some way by midwife.

Why did you decide to become a midwife?
I didn't so much as "decide" to become a midwife, instead I gradually grew into it.

What are your certifications and what do they mean?
I am licensed by the state of Florida. I completed a three year training program and sat for a 1 1/2 day licensing exam. We must complete certain CEU's [continuing education units] every 2 years for license renewal.

What should a client expect from you during the prenatal state?

I provide prenatal care on a normal schedule. Our prenatal care schedule is:

Every four weeks to 28 weeks gestation [period of development in the uterus, from conception to birth].
Then every two weeks until 36 weeks.
Then weekly until birth.

Under my license there is certain lab work required by the state. Other labs and ultrasounds are optional, and are discussed with clients. I like to emphasize having a healthy attitude, which includes diet, exercise, good lifestyle and mental health choices. I have completed several courses in alternative medicine. The alternative medicine courses I took were in:

Herbal medicine
Homeopathy
Stress reduction and relaxation
Ayurveda
Detoxification and healing
Naturopathy

This knowledge is often useful in assisting clients.

What should a client expect from you during labor and birth stages?

My main job in labor and delivery is to continually assess well-being and progress, and make suggestions as needed. Depending on the needs of the mother, I will also use what are now considered "doula" methods.

What should a client expect from you during the postpartum stage?

I visit the mother once or twice in the days soon after birth, telephone her at 9 or 10 days postpartum [the period shortly after childbirth], and see her at 6 wks postpartum.

What questions do you typically ask when interviewing a prospective client?

I first like to ascertain if she is a candidate for midwife care according to state rules. Then I ask about her reasons for considering home birth, and if she is willing to make the commitment to being healthy that is needed to maximize chances for normal delivery.

What are common misconceptions you hear from prospective parent(s)?

Because of the factory model of hospital births, and the fact that this style of birthing has now persisted so many years, there are many misconceptions - my mother's generation still knew that if they wanted to be safe through childbearing, they had to take responsibility to maintain good health. I think this attitude has largely been lost.

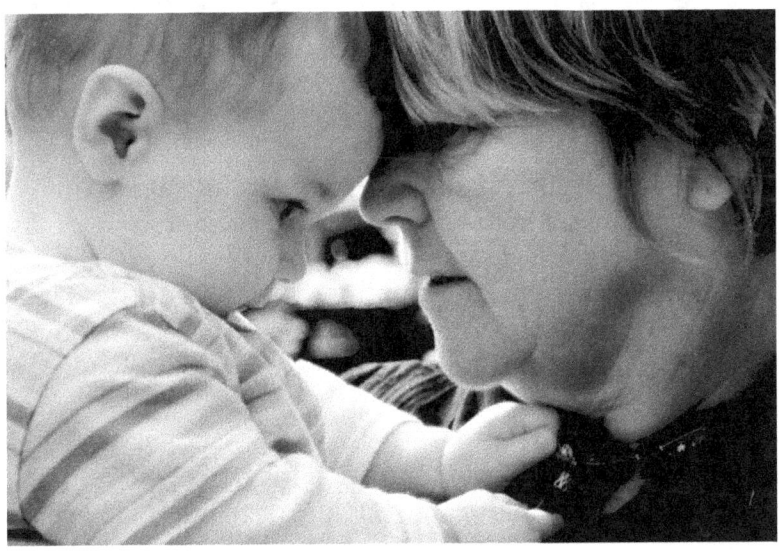

What are common questions you hear and how do you answer those questions?

Can we wait to cut the cord?
Can the father cut the cord?
What if there is cord around the neck?
Can we have a waterbirth?

-these I hear often.

Usually my clients have very good questions, but these are specific to to each client, and they will be answered to the best of my knowledge, and I will research the issue if needed.

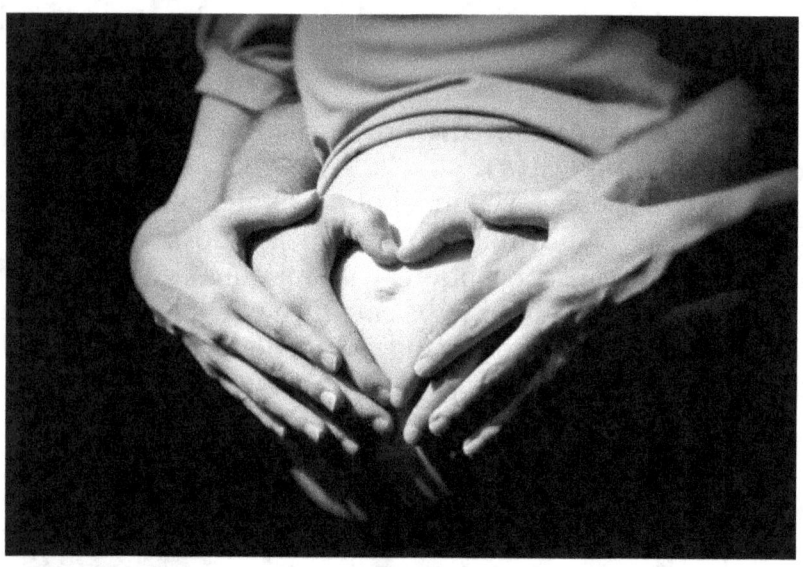

What is the single most important advice you wish to give new parents? Established parents?
Take the time to figure things out for yourself. Have confidence in your thinking ability. The internet is a useful tool, and a source of information. Unfortunately, it seems to promote an attitude that all solutions can be quickly obtained, rather than carefully considered.

What is your most memorable birthing experience?
I have had many memorable birth experiences. They are all an opportunity for learning, both those that were successful at home, and those that were not.

What are some memorable references / letters of gratitude you have received in your practice?
I have received many grateful letters. However I prefer to keep them to myself.

What other services do you offer?

Most clients actually find me through word of mouth. I also have a website, www.cathymatthewshomebirth.com

What is the fastest easiest way for a client to locate a Midwife?

Here in Florida, most midwives have websites, people can search 'midwives' in their city or area.

We also have the Florida Friends of Midwives website:

www.flmidwifery.blogspot.com

and

www.facebook.com/FLMidwifery

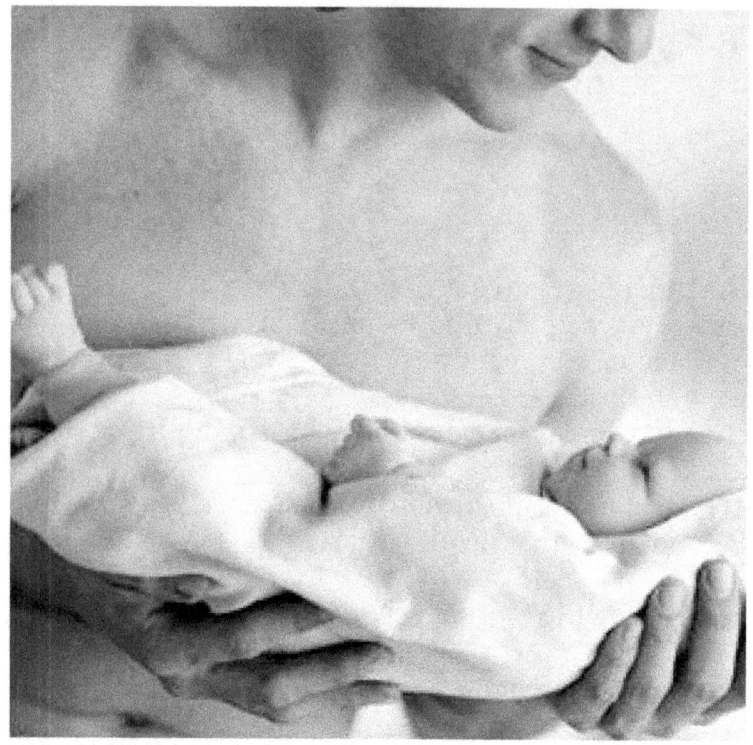

6 SUPPORT GROUP FOR DADS

Morning Star Women's Health & Birth Center

In this chapter, we have the opportunity to learn about a way that one Birthing Center helps new Dads-to-be cope with issues such as parenting roles, relationships, work and family balance, how to be more supportive, and what to expect during labor. By including this information, it is my hope that more birthing centers will want to provide a similar support group for their own Dads-to-be.

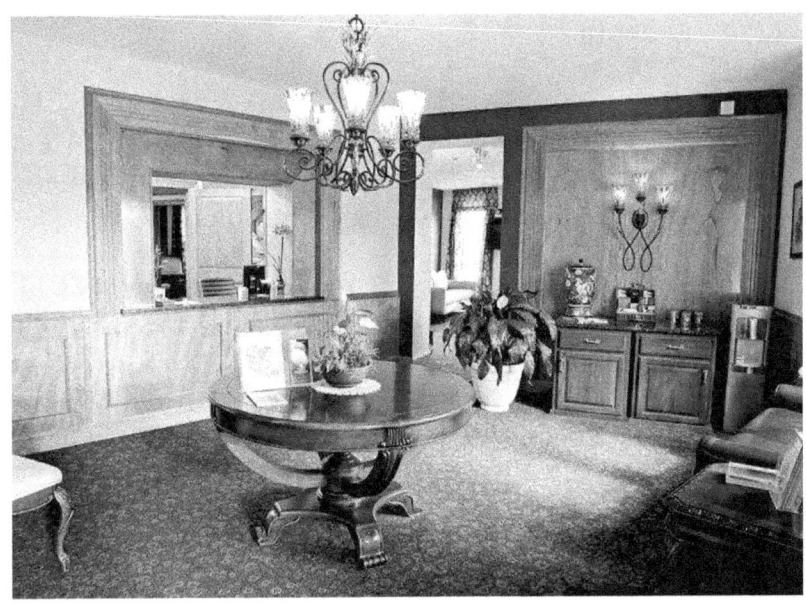

Morning Star Women's Health and Birth Center offers thorough well-woman and maternity care in the Midwives Model of Care. It is a woman-centered facility, that is focused on preparing and empowering families to make informed choices regarding their pregnancy.

"Our staff had a lovely feeling that the dads at Morning Star needed a safe space to discuss their own intense, delightful and meaningful experiences surrounding their pregnancies. Our clients are the center of our care, but we don't want their partners to feel like satellites; at the same time, the midwives and assistants may not be the best people to facilitate a fathers experience. From that, the Morning Star Dad's Group was born!" says Education and Community Outreach Coordinator, McKenna Keys.

As soon as a pregnant partner starts care at Morning Star, a dad is encouraged to join the support group. Currently, the group is open to ALL partners of pregnant people. They communicate with same-sex partners and non-traditional families that while this group has been historically male, and this may affect their participation, they are absolutely WELCOME to join.

A partner would want to join to share, validate, or learn from one another their thoughts about pregnancy, birth, and fatherhood. Dads are encouraged to share their challenges, invite feedback, and be supportive of other dads.

"We hope that those who participate are able to gain insight into their parenting practices and even some serenity, which may allow them to parent more effectively."

The dads group is still evolving. Right now, it is still very informal; it is being molded with the collaboration of "dad facilitators" and based on the feedback from the group. The group meets once a month, but with the interest they have been having, the frequency of meetings may need to be increased.

There is no registration or fee involved. Dads bring themselves, maybe snacks, and maybe a baby!

"We have an outline of topics and suggested prompts to use on a rotating basis, however, we encourage the facilitators to follow the flow of the group. As long as they are addressing the needs of the group, we are pleased to keep the structure relaxed. Dads are free to counsel one another, and also to ask our staff for support through our staff liaison. At the end of the meeting, the facilitators report how they felt the meeting went. We are looking at a more structured way to evaluate the meeting, but we also want to maintain the relaxed atmosphere."

The group meets specifically for the emotional and spiritual needs of the dads who are experiencing pregnancy and fatherhood. The facilitators are encouraged to bring any technical or physiologic questions to the staff liaison so that they can be answered appropriately.

It is a DADS ONLY group:

"Pregnant partners are not permitted because we want to preserve the sanctity of "dads time." It gives dads the chance to ask questions they might be nervous to broach with their partners."

"We encourage ALL partners of our clients to participate, particularly dads whose partners haven't delivered yet. Dads-to-be would particularly benefit from the experience of new dads because they get all sorts of validation and advice about how to support their partners in labor."

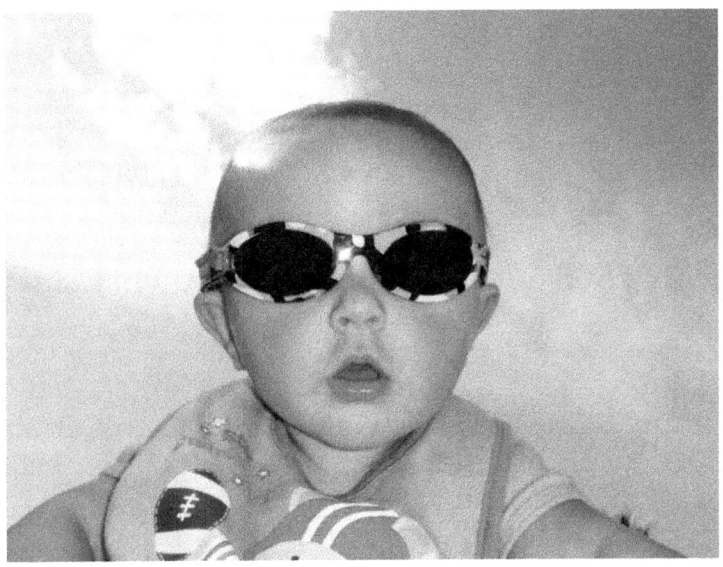

To learn more about the Morning Star Dad's Group, you may visit their website at www.morningstarbirth.com or you can call the center at 612-922-4784.

The BEST way to find out about it is to come to a meeting!

I asked McKenna if she is willing to assist / offer advice to readers who would like to see a Dad's group in their area/location, and she says she is always happy to take a phone call.

There are other classes available at Morning Star: "We are always adding new classes! Currently, some of our highlights include Bright Baby, Childbirth Preparation, Hypnobabies and Prenatal Yoga. Additionally we have two required classes, Handling Complications and Early Home Care. Coming to a free consultation is always a fantastic option and can be scheduled by phone."

Women's Health *and* Birth Center

To learn more about everything Morning Star Women's Center has to offer, visit www.morningstarbirth.com

Morning Star Women's Health and Birth Center
6111 Excelsior Boulevard
St. Louis Park MN 55416

Morning Star Women's Health and Birth Center
321 13th Street SE
Menomonie, WI 54751
715-231-3100

Facebook:
www.facebook.com/pages/Morning-Star-Womens-Health-and-Birth-Center/49037738302

email:
info@morningstarbirth.com

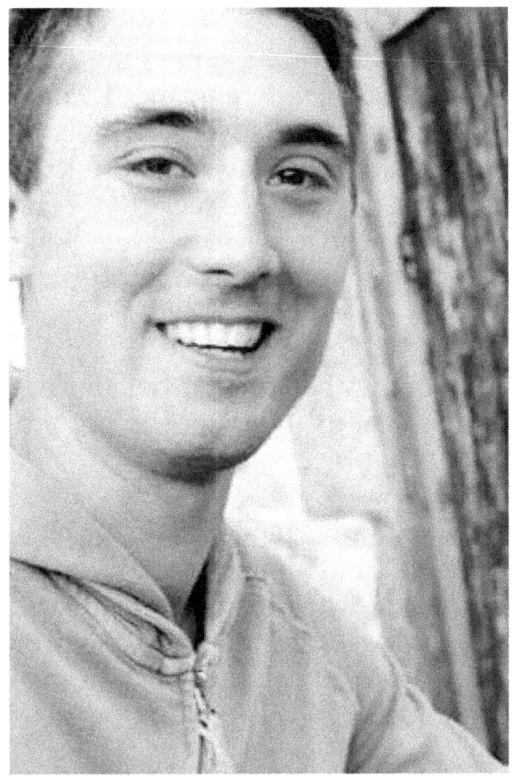

7 TRUST, RESPECT, AND COMFORT

Sean Hill

A Male Student Midwife's Perspective

My name is Sean Hill and I am a student midwife in the United Kingdom. I commenced my training in September 2010 and am now halfway through.

Being a midwife is so much more than helping somebody birth their baby. It involves a knowledgeable individual who the woman can trust, respect and be comfortable with throughout her pregnancy, the labour process and the postnatal period. My core values are to provide normality and to communicate well with women and their partners in order to promote health as well as providing informed choice.

Childbirth has always been something that has fascinated me. From a very young age I knew that I wanted to undertake this job. The reason why I love midwifery is because I am fascinated by pregnancy and labour and felt an overwhelming desire to be a part of that. I feel that I am a caring and considerate person who enjoys helping people and also, I wanted to break the mould and do a job that not many men do.

I wanted to work in healthcare, but did not want to work with sick or ill people, as pregnancy is not a disease and is a natural and beautiful process.

I always felt that my gender may pose an issue to me fulfilling my dream; but undeterred by negative words and attitudes from people who I respected and friends, I took the plunge, applied and was accepted into the programme. I had done some limited care experience back in my hometown, but actually providing care in this way was a new experience for me.

Males are not unheard of in midwifery in the United Kingdom; they make up less than 1% of all qualified midwives, however the number is now increasing. Most major hospitals in the United Kingdom have at least one male midwife, so many female midwives have worked with one. I find that the older generation of female midwives are neutral towards me, with some expressing a curiosity as to why I chose this career but it is the younger generation and the more newly qualified midwives that are very supportive and more willing to work with me.

Although the course is challenging, it is also extremely rewarding, learning all the processes involved and developing my existing knowledge base. The most challenging topics are understanding the mechanics of labour and to recognise the abnormal and deviations from the normal. My experience in practice has again been mixed; at times it is extremely stressful and difficult. One experience that I recall is when I had a major obstetric labour emergency that was unexpected and one minute the room was quiet with just me and the midwife present, and the next was full of midwives and doctors. I found it stressful; as I felt that I was useless and could not do anything except support the husband and reassure him, and keeping him updated on what was happening. Being a student, you feel that you don't know enough or that your input is undervalued. I felt like this in the beginning of my first year, that I did not know enough to be able to answer questions about certain issues. However, as I progressed through the first year, I realised I had learnt a lot and was able to apply my knowledge to practice. For example, I cared for a lady who was having problems with establishing breastfeeding. Having had lectures and practical sessions on positioning and attachment for the baby and mother, I was able to support and help the woman 'latch' the baby onto the breast successfully, using a hands off approach. It made me feel that I was sharing my gained knowledge with others for their benefit.

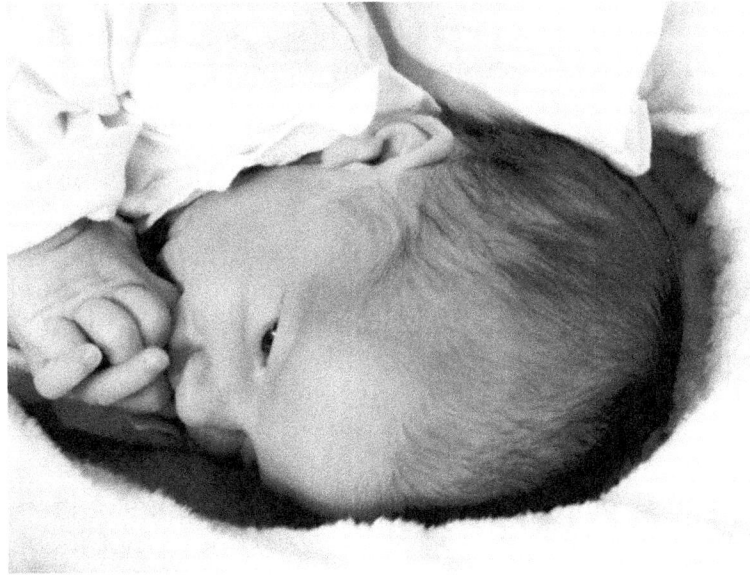

Upon starting my second year, I felt much more confident as I felt that I had made it past the first hurdle, and successfully passed my first year and things started to come more naturally to me; I felt like I knew what I was doing! I understood processes and along with extremely supportive coworkers, I felt extremely comfortable in my work environment.

Having a good relationship with your mentor(s) is key to being successful at the student level. You learn the most being out in practice, and it is important to constantly ask questions, knowing that you are supported by your mentor, who in turn teaches you all he/she knows. I have different mentors for each different department I work in. The departments are a community which consists of antenatal and postnatal appointments, antenatal ward, delivery suite and the birthing centre, postnatal ward and neonatal intensive care unit. I find all my mentors are willing to teach me; they tell me that I have great potential, which makes me feel even more confident, and increases my drive to succeed.

As previously mentioned, being a midwife is not just helping someone birth their baby; it is being an advocate for women throughout their pregnancy and a friendly face at appointments.

I would say that my favourite area to work, as is probably the same as many other midwives is in the delivery ward. I prefer low risk labour, which I define as women who labour who have no medical problems and have had an uneventful pregnancy with no interventions in the labour, and that they feel in control of the situation, are free and mobile; and I am a great believer in normality, with as little intervention as possible.

Although I understand that sometimes intervention is necessary and sometimes unavoidable, I believe that it is also too readily done in some instances. I believe that women should have the choice in all aspects of their pregnancy, in terms of pain relief and place of birth and I do believe that women should be informed antenatally of all aspects of labour and birth such as pain relief, place of birth, positions in labour and water therapy, as well as the complications, such as induction of labour or caesarean section. I also think it is good for women to have a birth plan in place for labour, but also for them to be aware that it may not go to plan due to unforeseen complications in labour, and not to be disappointed if they did not achieve the birth they desired [Birth plans that I have seen, which women have written themselves, contain details of where they would like to give birth, what pain relief they would like to try or avoid, who will be present and what they would like post delivery].

Whenever I am caring for a woman in labour along with a qualified midwife, I always feel so privileged, as it is an extremely intimate time and they are willing to share it with me.

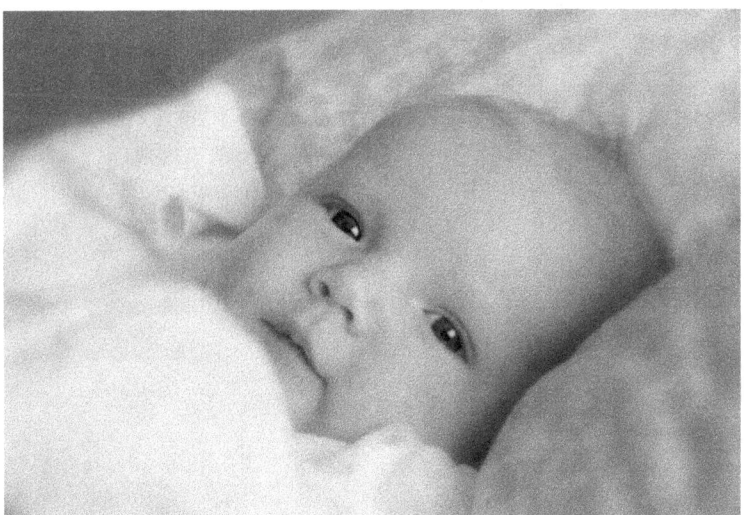

The most important advice I would give to a woman is to believe in herself that she can do it and not be scared or stressed as this can slow down the labour; breathe through the contractions and pain, and keep your mind on what the outcome is.

My advice to anyone wanting to join this wonderful career is, if you feel extremely strong about midwifery, then definitely consider applying, as it is one of the most rewarding and amazing career choices. Everyday I am so pleased that I embarked on this journey. Although I still have far to go in terms of knowledge and personal development, I am excited as to where this will take me in the years to come.

Sean Hill is a Student Midwife in the {south of England} UK. He will graduate in 2013 as a registered midwife (RM). If you'd like to learn more about his experience as a Student Midwife, feel free to email him at:
studentmidwifesean@hotmail.co.uk

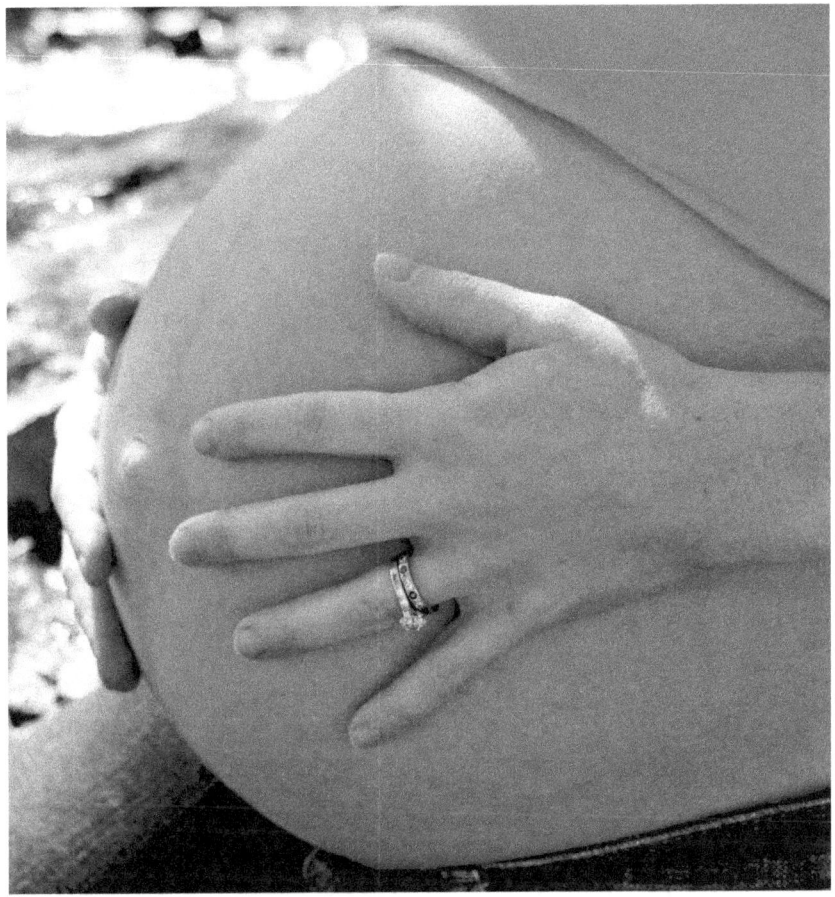

8 MANAGING ACHES & PAINS

How can a Birth Ball help you?

Pregnancy brings with it back aches, acid indigestion, restlessness, sore and swollen feet, sleep issues and more. During pregnancy, a womans posture suffers greatly because of the increased strain placed on her back [not to mention the rest of her body]. One way to help mom get through her pregnancy much easier, is by the use of what's known as a Birth Ball. In this chapter I will explain two different types.

But first, a cute story from Keith Roberts about them:

Sixteen years ago [1998], when I first started attending births, there were no birth balls in my local three hospitals. So I always took my own.

I remember at one of those first births, having the nurse (who was busy typing in front of the monitor) ask me what the ball was called.

I said "We doulas call it a birth ball." She needed to enter its name into the record since it was being used by the laboring mother.

And later, several nurses came into the room and took turns sitting and bouncing and giggling on the birth ball! It was their first encounter with the big ball.

I guess there is a first time for everything, and I can still remember their delight.

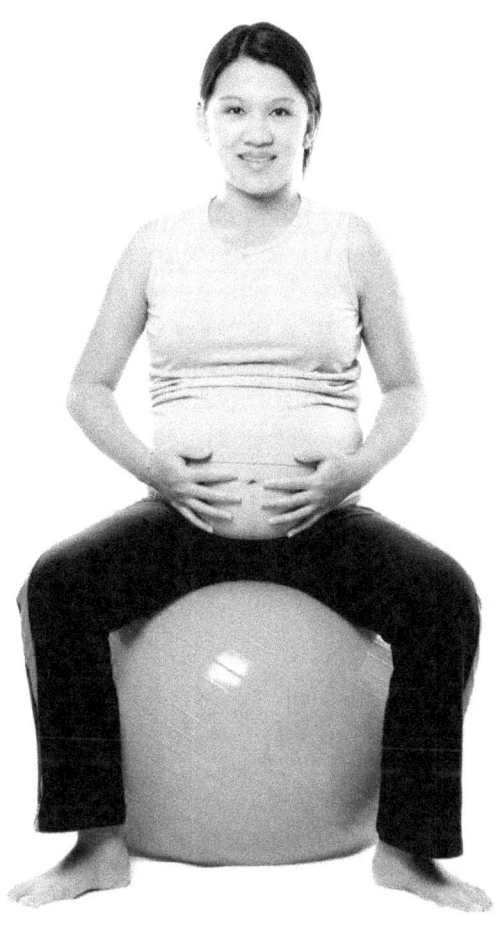

The use of a birth ball can help speed the labor and delivery process, and reduce the need for an episiotomy; it can assist in the decent of the baby into the birth canal as well. The use of a birth (aka 'fitness') ball will help a woman who is pregnant to maintain proper posture and increase her overall core stability. A birth ball is used in a variety of ways to alleviate aches and pains. Sitting on the birth ball at any time, but especially during pregnancy, helps relieve the strain on your hips and low back by forcing you to engage your abdominal muscles and sit with good posture. It can prove to be more comfortable for mom than a chair or bed. Additionally, the ball is easier for mom to get onto, and to rise from, than the couch, floor, or chair-simply by shifting her weight forward and rolling onto her feet. By positioning mom's body in certain ways, it can also help the baby turn his/her body [kneeling over the ball can ease back strain and encourage the baby to settle into an optimal position]. A woman can lightly bounce on it, or gently rock back and forth or side to side, to decrease perineal pressure. She can also lean over the ball, allowing the baby to hang down, in order to decrease any back pain or back labor. Gentle exercise on the birthing ball can strengthen the abdominal "pushing" muscles, as well as the lower-back muscles that minimize back pain.

The ball can also be used to rest in a relaxed position, and to faciliate massage by a doula or dad. During labor, the birth ball (also sometimes referred to as a birthing ball) really provides support and eases discomfort.

And once you've had your baby and your provider has given you the OK to begin working out, and you feel you are ready to get back into shape, your birthing ball is great for postpartum exercises. So starting early in the pregnancy with the birthing ball is a good idea!

You will need to decide, based on your height and comfort level, which size is best for you. Check to make sure it's the right fit for you by sitting directly on top, with your feet flat on the floor. Make sure that your legs are at a 90 degree angle (if your knees are too high it may cause strain on your hips).

Your midwife or doula probably has one or two as well and can assist you with choosing the correct size for home use. For an average woman of 5'5" it will probably be the 65cm ball, if you are shorter than 5'5", you will want to see if the smaller 55 cm size works better. A taller woman will want to choose the larger 75cm size.

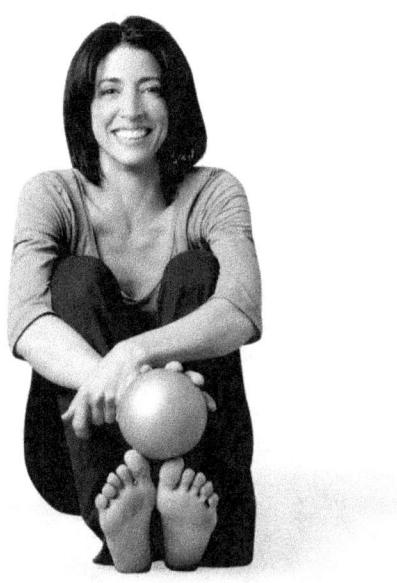

A newer type of ball [to help alleviate pain and increase relaxation] are Miracle Balls, created by a former dancer named Elaine Petrone. These are much smaller than the traditional birth ball previously mentioned, but they are providing relief for many pregnant women. She created the Miracle Ball Method to heal herself after she suffered a career-ending injury. After her own high-risk pregnancy (with twins!) she developed The Miracle Ball Method (specifically) for Pregnancy. It is a program designed to help women deal with the pains, stress and physical changes caused by pregnancy. The boxed set includes the illustrated book and two rather 'squishy' and small 'miracle balls' which can provide a great deal of relief for a pregnant mom, including the postpartum stage to regain her shape back. The kit allows muscles to relax and become supple enough to allow the body to realign and reshape.

How do they work?

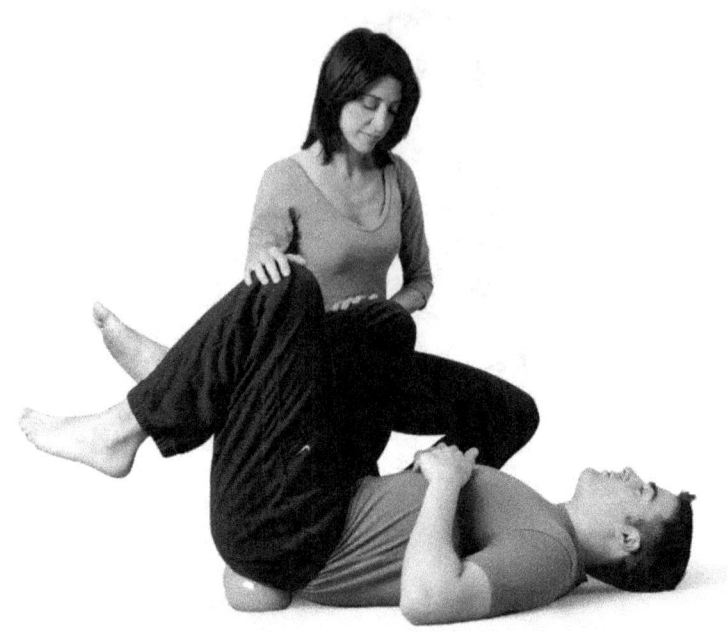

Let's say for example that you have a sore back. By resting your aching back on these squishy grapefruit-sized balls and letting your body sink into them, you are essentially unworking the muscles that hurt. Elaine shows how proper breathing works in conjunction with a range of low-impact ways to use the Miracle Balls to provide relief from head to toe.

The program incorporates breathing techniques that focus on exhalations to strengthen the diaphragm and relieve anxiety and fatigue. There are movements for specific problem areas, as well as moves for the entire body, and variations to use in later months (when it is no longer advised for mom to lie flat on her back). The final exercises can help reshape the body after birth. The book also addresses labor, breastfeeding, and baby-carrying issues.

Elaine is helping thousands of people conquer pain, stress, and injury with her range of products and live workshops. She also trains students at hospitals and healing centers across the country. You may want to see if she will be hosting a class in your area.

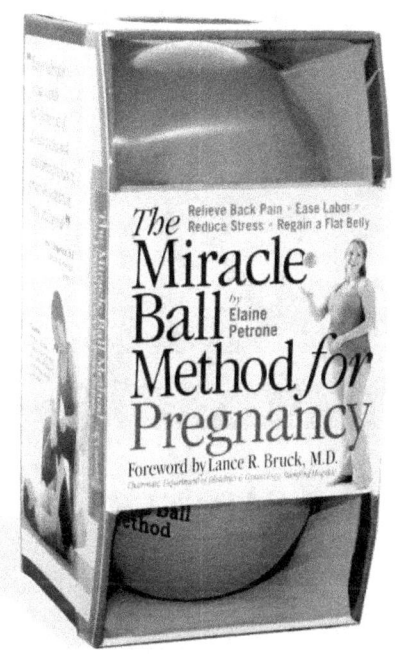

The Miracle Ball Method for Pregnancy is Elaine's third book, developed for prenatal and postpartum women to help relieve back pain, ease labor, reduce stress, and re-gain a flat belly. Her specially designed soft (grapefruit-sized) ball is formulated with just the right amount of "give". When mom rests her body on the ball, it is supportive yet not too spongy, nor too inflexible.

For more information about Elaine's products, classes, and blog, visit her website at www.elainepetrone.com

You may also want to head over to Amazon to learn more about this specific kit for pregnant women.

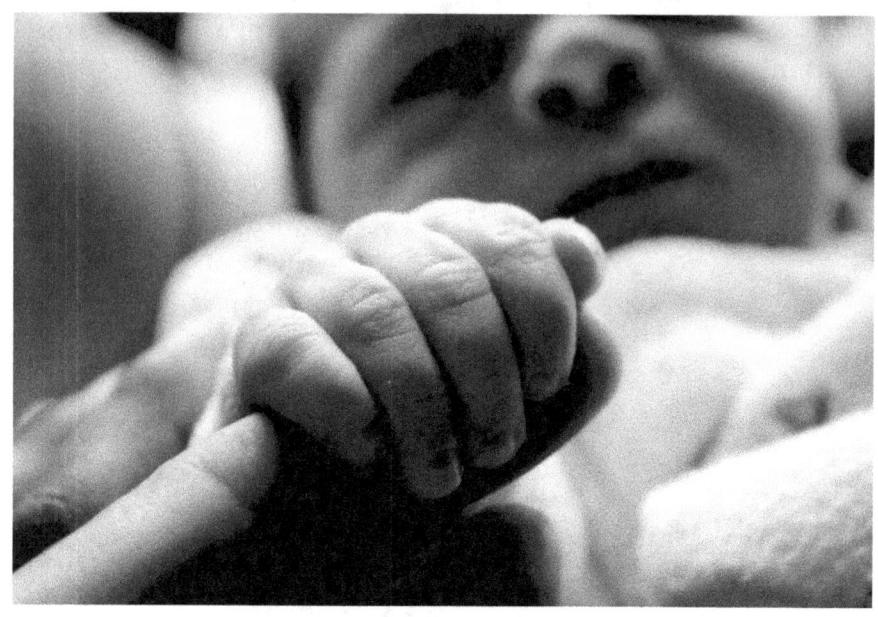

9 FOR DADS AND PARTNERS

I know you are super excited about your baby (or babies?!) coming soon. But I'll bet you're scared too. In a different way than your spouse is. There is a lot of focus on the woman of course, because she is going to be enduring the actual pain of childbirth. You can take the time to learn about all the stages of pregnancy, labour and delivery, and how to bond with your newborn; but obviously you cannot know exactly what it feels like to carry and birth a newborn. So, you may start having doubts about how you will be able to handle it all. What many people [especially those who have never hired a midwife or doula] don't consider is that the dad or partner in the delivery room has his/her own issues as well. I would like to strongly suggest that you at least TRY to set those uncomfortable thoughts aside. Did you know that men who are present at their child's birth, are more likely to get and stay involved in the care and nurturing of them?

You may not realize this but years ago, men weren't even allowed in the delivery room. Guys had to 'wait' in the waiting room, pacing as they waited for their offspring to be sprung. Today, however, about 90 percent of dads are taking a hands-on approach in the birthing process. I'm personally elated about this!

Dr. Robert Bradley wrote the book Husband-Coached Childbirth (in 1974), in which he empowered men to take as crucial a role in the birthing process as possible. At the time, Bradley was both hailed as a champion for men's rights to be in the delivery room, but also criticized as someone who was trying to advocate controlling women. This book 'gave birth' to the 'Bradley method'; in fact there are classes still running today in the US based on this method.

Sure there are all sorts of things you'll need to figure out and plan for such as choosing nursery furniture, going through tons of names for your baby, and taking Lamaze or other classes with your spouse. But guys, I'll bet you may still feel out of place when attending the birth of your child.

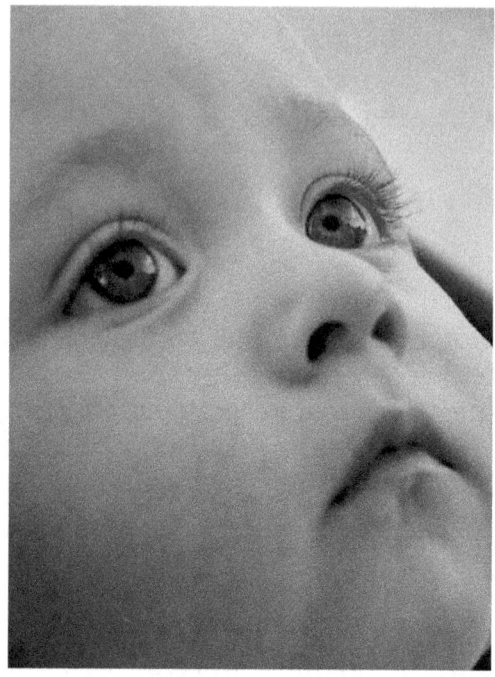

So what do you believe you should do? You've probably heard the horror stories about being called every name in the book and being clawed, scratched, bitten and blamed for every single issue on the planet. It can be difficult watching someone you love in pain, and I will tell you this: childbirth is definitely painful.

In this section, I'm going to give you advice on the best way (in my opinion) you can prepare for your baby, and help your woman. I hope you utilize these and I hope mom thanks you profusely for doing so.

DO NOT RUN AWAY.

When you are with your woman in the delivery room, being as supportive as possible, you are more than likely reducing her need for pain medication, reducing her stress level, increasing her satisfaction with the whole birth experience, and increasing her confidence in herself as a mom. There is however the possibility that your partner might not want you present throughout her labour and birth, perhaps because she doesn't want you to see her in childbirth. It is very important then that you two talk through these issues during the pregnancy to avoid problems once labor begins. You may even talk with other guys about their experiences in the delivery room, but keep in mind that everyone is different and one guy's experience may not be the same as yours. Of course if she absolutely wants you there with her, then, you have no choice in the matter, do you?

By arranging to have a midwife and / or doula present then, if it all turns out to be too much, you can leave the room for a short break. Be sure to make it a really short break though, and not during the end stage of labour!

What a woman needs most when she is in labour is to feel safe and secure.

Be prepared to make decisions. Only you and your partner know what you both want, but she may not be in the best condition to make the tough decisions-so please be ready to step in if the situation calls for it.

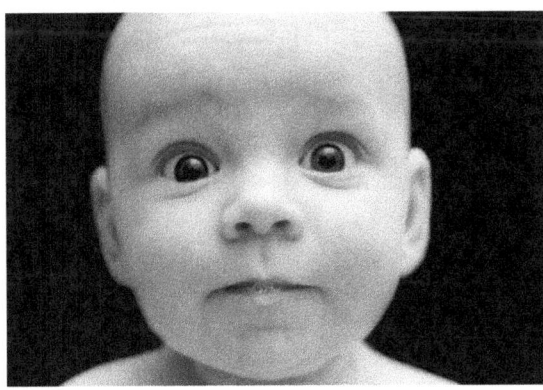

With the help of your midwife or doula, you will have rehearsed beforehand where and how to massage mom especially when she is having a contraction. Make sure to have practiced, well enough in advance, breathing techniques and other comfort measures.

BACKPACK/TRAVEL BAG / LABOUR KIT

Make sure that you have your car gassed up, and mechanically 'ready'.

Labor takes a long time, normally anywhere from 12 to 18 hours, perhaps even longer (one of mine was 44 hours). Most of the time labor takes place at night, so it is imperative that you, dad, be comfortable too. I highly recommend that you pack these items before the due date; ask your midwife or doula for suggestions as well:

An extra shirt and/or change of clothes for yourself and toothpaste, toothbrush, deodorant, mouthwash.

A bathing suit or shorts, in case you want to join your partner in the bath or shower.

Have a big zippered bag of snacks handy for yourself.

A tennis ball to help alleviate back labor pains (or the balls I mentioned in the previous chapter!).

A CD or cassette player to set the mood in the room-which she may or may not want after all-ask.

Candles for soft lighting. Be sure to bring scented (her favourite scents) and non-scented (in case she can't stand the smell at the moment).

Things to do for both of you: cards, board games, crossword puzzles, etc for the early stages of labor.

Bring lollipops for her to suck on in case she gets hungry.

Bring a camera. But I must warn you. Don't snap pictures, or let anyone else do so for that matter, unless you have gotten express permission from mom **at that very moment**...

Bring lots of change (actual coins-get your piggy bank started ahead of time for this purpose) for the vending machine items you may feel you 'need'.

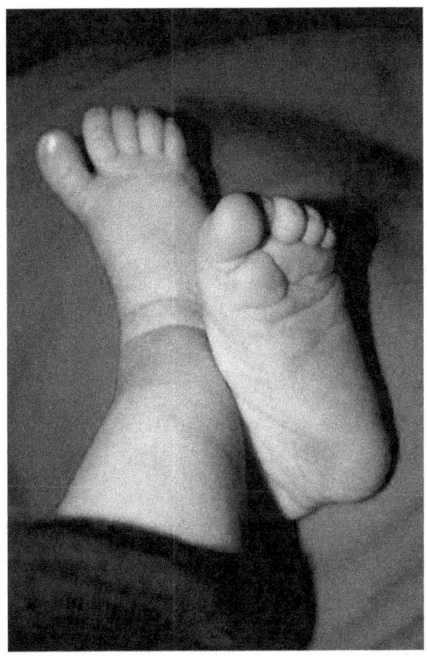

Bring your list of phone numbers for the people that you will want to call shortly after your baby is here. You will be asked for the time of delivery, number of hours in labour, sex of the baby, birth weight, height / length in inches, and how mom and baby are doing. So, write these things down (on the notepad you bring) before making your calls. Or, better yet, designate one person beforehand to take your call, and have that person call your 'list' for you.

COVERED DISH

Weird title I know, but basically, one of the best ways you can help mom is to have established before-hand, a list of friends or family, who have agreed to drop off (leave it at your doorstep) one or two meals per day after the baby is born. It is going to be very difficult for her to move around and she will be very hungry, especially if she is breastfeeding or expressing milk. She will not have time nor energy to freshen up and visit with guests-your baby will be hungry often so mom will need to be able to breastfeed or pump milk easily and quickly (and thus may be walking around the house in PJ's and other comfy clothes for a long while).

The supportive and helpful friend/family member can chitchat with you dad, at the door, hand you the dish, and then be on their merry way. The dish they bring should be pre-cooked, and have a short hand-written note including the temperature to set the oven [or microwave] for, and how long it should be re-heated to be perfect.

I will list a few recipe names here that you may want to ask someone to prepare. You can always look online for recipes that you two are particularly fond of, and create a list, then send each to a person on your list using the online sharing tool/icon that is usually present near the title of the recipe. This way, you can send the exact one you want to the person's inbox. If that's too much work, just make a list, like below, and ask who is willing to provide help and support in this way after baby is born. It would be a great idea to use a calendar and write in each 'box' who is bringing what, and then keep that posted on your fridge so you can look forward to your visitor's presence and the delicious (hopefully LOL) meal they will furnish. Use this calendar later to hand-write and send thank-you cards too. OK, here you go:

CHILI
LASAGNA
TAKE OUT CHINESE OR THAI ENTREES, RICE, etc.
PASTA SALAD
POT PIE (beef, chicken, lamb-your choice)
COBB SALAD
GARDEN SALAD
FRESH FRUIT (peeled/diced/sliced and chilled)
MACARONI & CHEESE
COBBLER (apple, cherry, blueberry-your choice)
MEATBALLS (and spaghetti, or with makings for Subs)
PIZZA
MEATLOAF
TURKEY TETRAZZINI
BISCUITS
COFFEE CAKE
COOKIES
PIE
FRESH VEGGIES (sliced/diced/chilled with dip)

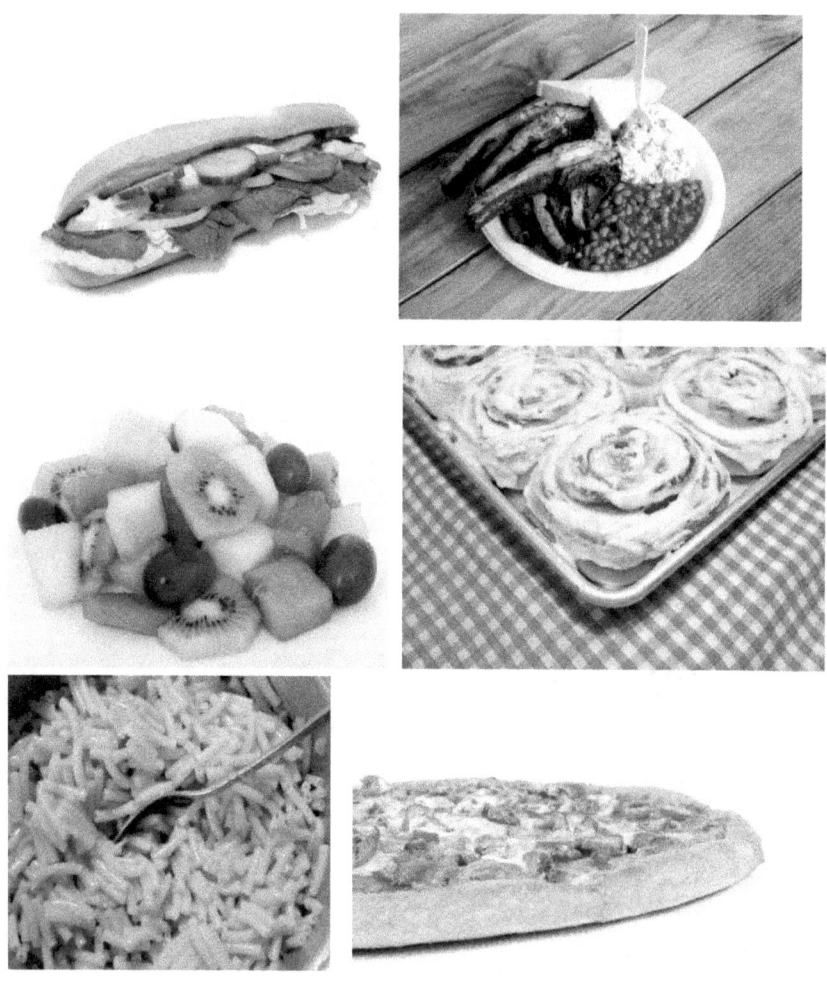

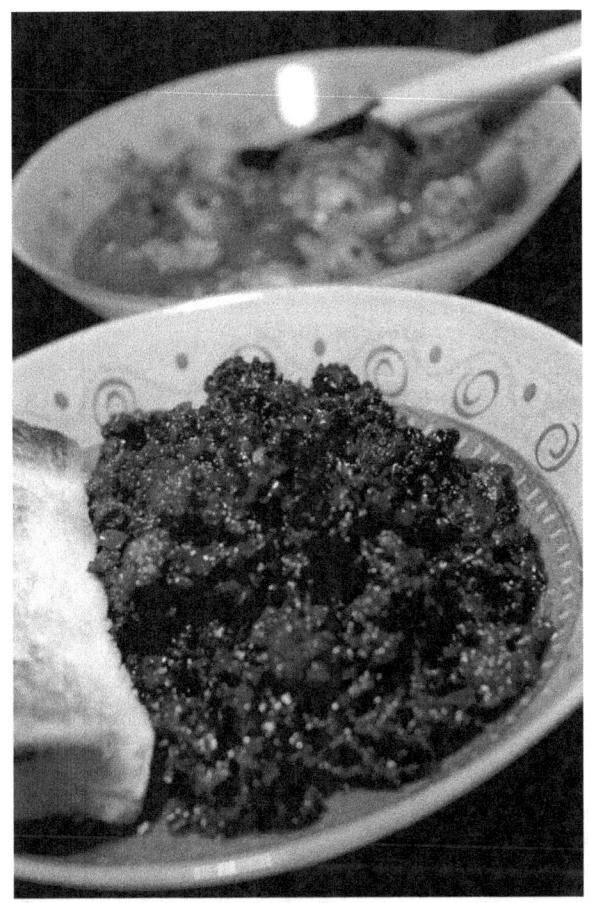

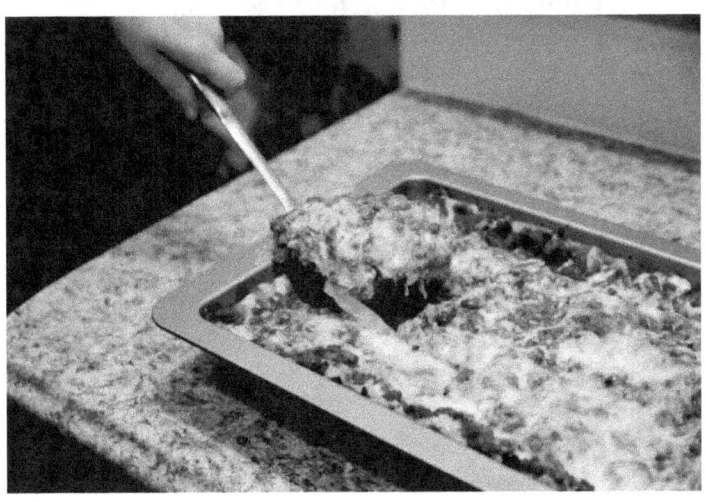

(Did that make you hungry?)

And if you're not sure how to ask, here is a short quick note you can send out via email, or phone call:

Dear Friend/Family Member,

Would you be so kind as to provide a meal or two, after the baby is born, when we are home recuperating and taking care of our dear baby?

We are going to be very tired, and not able to properly feed ourselves, let alone freshen up for guests. It would be wonderful if you could swing by on a given date, and drop something delicious at our door, to help replenish us.

If you are willing and able to do so, I will send you a recipe soon and provide more info before our due date. We thank you from the bottom of our hearts for being so giving and considerate of our new family.

You can of course tweak that if you wish!

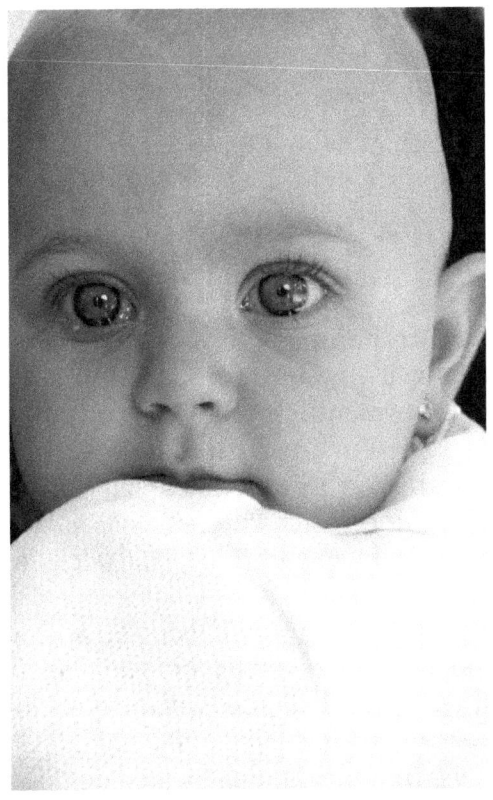

Do not forget that your sole purpose at being in the birthing room with mom is to provide strength and support.

She will suffer considerable anxiety over the delivery, especially if it is her first time. She may have taken birthing classes with you alongside her, and she may have been told what it is going to be like by a multitude of different people, but until she actually experiences it for herself, she will be apprehensive.

Once the baby is here, ask Mom what she needs for you to do. Does she want you to start calling your list of people, or does she just want you to stay by her side and sleep – or what? Help her relax. She may still want a massage or back rub, and she'll still be feeling some pain. Above all, enjoy the moment and get as much rest as you can.

You will want to pamper mom at this point. She has been through a lot physically and emotionally; it would be a good time to show her how much you love and appreciate her. You may have asked someone to bring flowers (that you picked out beforehand for this occasion), pack her favourite chocolates, hand-write a love note while she rests. Whatever you decide to do, find a truly special way to mark this occasion.

As the caring partner that you are, you will want to actively take part in the job of parenting; and that means sharing in the baby-care duties as much as mom wants you to--even at night.

Your role is very important.

Your physical presence and emotional strength will mean a great deal to mom's feelings of security. And mom will always remember everything you did to support her through labor and birth. Reassure her on a continuous basis, that you are going to be with her every step of the way.

Congratulations.

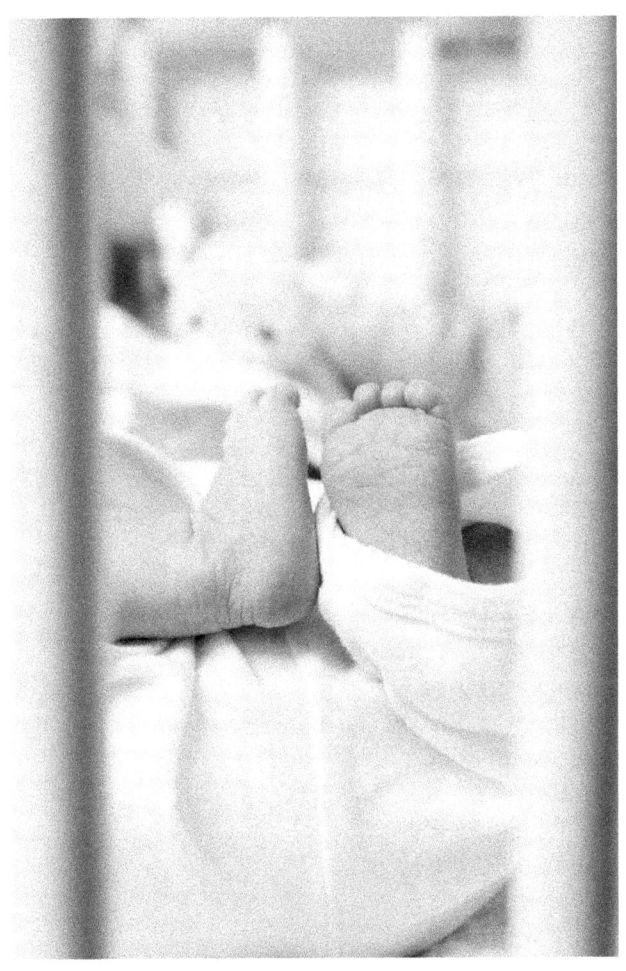

THE END

REFERENCES

For more information on how to get transparency from your local hospitals and doctors, see www.thebirthsurvey.com

Henci Goer
The Thinking Woman's Guide to a Better Birth

Robert Bradley
Husband-Coached Childbirth (Fifth Edition): The Bradley Method of Natural Childbirth

Elaine Petrone
The Miracle Ball Method for Pregnancy: Relieve Back Pain, Ease Labor, Reduce Stress, Regain a Flat Belly

How to find a Midwife and Doula, in the pursuit of a more natural childbirth experience
[ebook version is available at Amazon.com]

PHOTOGRAPHS / IMAGES
Cover image: Martine Lemmens
Cover design: Petra Ortiz
Acknowledgements: Justyna Furmanczyk www.janedoephoto.co.uk
Introduction: Keith Roberts
Keith Roberts pages: 1,9,11,14,15,19, 29, 34
Kelly Burnett, page 24
Mari Carmen Guinovart, page 26
Cathy Matthews, page 37
Emily Cahal, page 40
Petra Ortiz page 39, 42, 55,76
Mckenna Keys, page 43, 46
Vincent Valentino, page 45
Sean Hill: page 47
Guenter M. Kirchweger, page 49
Olga Doroschenkova, page 51
Roberta Lott, page 53
Elaine Petrone www.elainepetrone.com pg 57, 58,59

Daniel Forero, page 60
Neco Garnica, page 62
Sam Hatch & Erin Lee, page 63
Sandi Brubaker, page 65
Food page 68:
Ove Tøpfer
Chris Cummings www.iwdonline.com
Hotel in Eastbourne www.eastbourneguide
Luis Solis
Stephanie
Food Page 69:
Nathalie Dulex
Jim O'Connor
Catalin Pop, page 71
Jean Scheijen | www.vierdrie.nl page 73

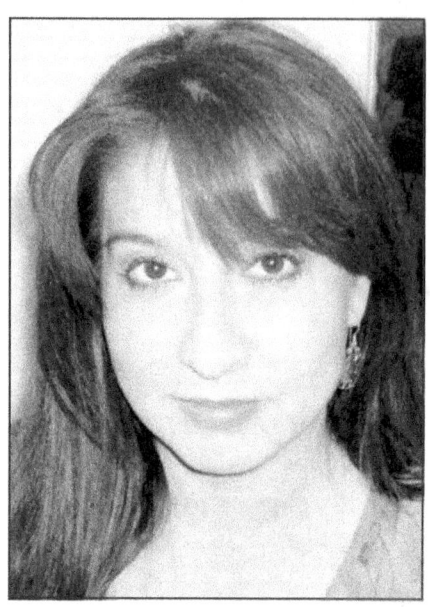

From the Author

Thank you for taking the time to learn more about the roles of Midwives and Doulas in your pursuit of a more natural childbirth experience. Feel free to contact them for more information and assistance.

Did you enjoy what you read? If so, please let me know: http://amazon.com/author/petra

Petra

www.ingramcontent.com/pod-product-compliance
Lightning Source LLC
Chambersburg PA
CBHW072339290526
45794CB00002B/935